The
Researcher
Experience
in
Qualitative
Research

We dedicate this book to our parents,
Joseph J. and Irene A. Diemert
and
Francis and Wanda Gutowski,
who instilled in us the value of education and learning,
coupled with great respect for our own and others' life
experiences

PART 1

Researcher Experiences With Various Populations and in Different Settings

---

Introduction: What About the Researcher Experience?

Susan Diemert Moch

Marie F. Gates

We have wrestled with what we should do with the researcher experience since our early beginnings in qualitative research. In graduate school, we could talk about our experience with other students in research seminars. And through graduate school presentations, we could easily share our research experience with our cohorts. More recently, presenting at some research conferences has provided opportunities for continued processing of the researcher experience. However, the more we have progressed in our respective research careers, the more we have realized the importance the researcher experience has to the findings of the research. The researcher experience is not just peripheral to the research and should thus have a place in the reporting of the research. We think it is time the researcher experience be given more prominence than just a discussion in doctoral seminars and as an add-on in presentations at some research conferences.

This book emerged from our ponderings about what to do with the researcher experience. Our intent in this book is to raise the issue of the researcher experience and to encourage further discussion about what to do with the researcher experience.

We address the following questions:

1. Why is discussing the researcher experience important?
2. What are the similarities and differences with the researcher experience across disciplines?
3. Are there circumstances in which reporting the researcher experience is more important than others?
4. What does a researcher do with the researcher experience?
5. How has the researcher experience been reported?
6. What possibilities exist or can be created to share the researcher experience?

We are excited that Sage Publications welcomed our proposal for this book in our first discussion with them. In earlier ventures regarding the research experience, Moch met some resistance to including the research experience (Moch, 1988, 1989, 1990, 1992). The interest and enthusiasm shown by Sage Publication editors, colleagues at the 1998 Qualitative Health Research Conference, and researchers from several disciplines have convinced us of the need for this book.

We shared the literature review on the researcher experience through an evocative poster presentation at the Qualitative Health Research Conference (Moch & Gates, 1998). Through discussions with colleagues at the conference, we became even more aware of the need for further dialogue on the researcher experience. Conference participants were anxious to read the citations we shared through our poster presentation, just as they were keenly interested in how the researcher experience was reported in books and in journals. Students from various disciplines were particularly interested in having a place to discuss the meaning of the researcher experience and the ways to process it. More experienced qualitative researchers noted the need to have a forum to explore ways to discuss pros and cons of the inclusion of the researcher experience, in both oral and written ways.

When we approached researchers from several disciplines about this book, we received enthusiastic support. We found great interest in authoring chapters, as many colleagues, like us, had wondered what to do with the researcher experience. The book has provided them a forum for sharing their experiences.

Our hope for this book is to promote dialogue and reflection around questions related to the researcher experience. We do not propose definitive answers nor offer suggestions applicable to all disciplines. We intend to raise awareness of the issue of the researcher experience and to offer change possibilities for what to do with the researcher experience. It is our hope that future researchers will know how to process the researcher experience and how to share it. In addition, we hope publishers will open avenues for sharing the researcher experience. We want the researcher experience to be used in teaching, analyzing, and reporting research.

The book includes three sections. The section titled "Researcher Experiences With Various Populations and in Different Settings" brings together research on breast cancer, as discussed by Moch in the health care arena, and research on sensitive issues, such as victimizing sexualization, addressed by Smith in the third chapter. The authors describe concerns dealt with throughout the research experience. In addition, the section includes researcher experience issues with families and communities and in an organizational context. The chapter by Gates and Lackey describes issues of concern for researchers in working with families and children. The ongoing program of research in communities, as described by Zerwekh and the St. Louis team in Chapter 5, provides examples of continued reflection on research in the community. In the sixth chapter, Elsbach gives examples of the range of organizational researcher interviews.

The second section, "Processing the Researcher Experience," enumerates various ways to process the researcher experience. In Chapter 7, Moch and Cameron describe an interview procedure for dealing with the researcher experience. The issues of gender orientation, cross-cultural concerns, and mentoring are discussed in the next chapter, by Simmons, Gates, and Thompson. Then Gates and Hinds discuss team processing in research. Last, Ochberg, a psychologist, reflects on his own processing in interviewing and analyzing data, in Chapter 10.

"Reporting the Researcher Experience," the third section, includes suggestions for reporting the research experience. In Chapter 11, Moch provides examples of researcher experiences published in books, journals, and other areas. Suggestions for reporting the research experience are enumerated by Moch and Gates in Chapter 12. The last two chapters, then, provide examples of how the research experience can be reported in the disciplines of sociology and religious studies, respectively. In Chapter 13, Pierce describes research on gender-related research and how her experience was an integral part of the research. And last, Gross, an experienced and well-published researcher in religious studies, provides examples of how she has integrated the researcher experience into her research program, in Chapter 14.

REFERENCES

Moch, S. D. (1988). *Health in illness: Experiences with breast cancer.* Unpublished doctoral dissertation, University of Minnesota, Minneapolis.

Moch, S. D. (1989). Health within illness: Conceptual evolution and practice possibilities. *Advances in Nursing Science, 11*(4), 23-31.

Moch, S. D. (1990). Health within the experience of breast cancer. *Journal of Advanced Nursing, 15,* 1426-1435.

Moch, S. D. (1992, April). *Incorporating the research experience into the research report.* Paper presented at Midwest Nursing Research Conference, Chicago, IL.

Moch, S. D., & Gates, M. F. (1998, February). *Reporting the researcher experience.* Poster session presented at the Qualitative Health Research Conference, Edmonton, Canada.

2

The Researcher Experience in Health Care Research

Susan Diemert Moch

My experience as a researcher in qualitative research has been a source of great reflection, inner struggle, and ethical questioning. Some of the difficulty occurred because of my being a nurse as well as a researcher. At times, I wondered if I was first a nurse and then a researcher or first a researcher and then a nurse. Sometimes, the difficulty arose because of my experience as a mother, wife, midlife woman, or professor. In other words, the researcher experience and all the reflection and struggle happened, in part, because of who I am. And I don't want to change that.

What I do want to change is what we do with the researcher experience. I want to talk about the researcher experience openly, to share the researcher experience in conference presentations and in publications. I would like researchers to struggle together with questions and concerns related to the researcher experience. I would like the knowledge emerging from the researcher experience to be available to others. With these goals in mind, I will share some of my experiences with research in health care. In this chapter, seven major issues emanating from the researcher experience are discussed, and examples from health care research are used for illustration.

ISSUES RELATED TO THE
RESEARCHER EXPERIENCE

Intimate Discussion

Little prompts more intimate discussion than having a midlife nurse researcher ask a midlife research participant to tell what it is like to have breast cancer. The women participants in my studies (Moch, 1990, 1995, 1998) were happy to tell their stories and through the telling, have someone validate their respective experiences with breast cancer. The women told about their fear of death, their feelings about their bodies, their reflections about life, and their concerns about not being alive for their children's future birthdays.

These intimate conversations affected me. After the intimate encounters with the women in my studies, I would try to put my thoughts on tape. I would try to write what I thought in my journal, and I would often reflect on what I thought about what they said. Sometimes, I wrote poetry about what happened during the experience of the interview. But most often, I needed to talk to someone about my experience. That someone was usually my husband and sometimes my sister or a friend.

How would it feel not to have a breast? How important is a breast in my own sexuality? What must it be like to be so sick from chemotherapy that you can hardly discuss a prom, a sporting event, a class, or even a graduation party with your child? How would the people I love react to my having breast cancer? Most important, how would I live my life with the news these women were given?

When I was not thinking about my own reaction to breast cancer, I was often in awe about how these women were dealing with their situations. I often pondered, given the circumstance, how can this woman do so well? I marveled at the love the women were shown by family and friends. I could not believe the openness of the women in sharing their experiences.

Participant or Patient

Another issue in health care research is whether the person in the research is first a patient or client or a research participant. Discourse on whether the nurse researcher is the nurse or the researcher when interviewing individual participants, groups, or communities is common in the nursing literature. When participants know that the researcher is a nurse, questions and comments directed to persons in a nurse role often emerge. Many researchers have taken the stand that the nurse researcher is first a nurse and then a researcher. So if someone's health is in danger or if someone needs information for a health decision, the nurse researcher will be the nurse. However, if the issue is not of a critical nature or if the traditional nurse response would decrease the sharing of the participant's experience, researchers have supported a more traditional research interview approach. I acknowledge that I cannot separate the researcher role from my nurse role and have in fact referred to myself as a researcher-practitioner, wherein both roles are valued and recognized on an equal level in my work. I argue I can't be otherwise.

Participant or Friend

My research with women diagnosed with breast cancer has involved many contacts with participants. Initially, I met with the participants two times (Moch, 1990), and then 5 years later, I interviewed the same women again (Moch, 1998). Partly because of my involvement with the women over time and partly because of the intimate nature of our conversations, I got to know the participants quite well. One participant called me after our interview and said there was something she did not talk about very much in the interview that she thought was important for me to know, so she wanted to schedule another interview. This woman was very candid about her experiences and very artistic in her expression. She was, like me, a graduate student at the time of our initial interviews. Even though her discipline was different from mine, we both had read and thought about many of the same issues. We had an immediate connection during our interviews. I often wondered how this affected my research process and the reporting of my findings. I did realize that when I was using an example from the research to illustrate a theme, her words often emerged in my mind. Also, the woman was the first woman of the participants that I knew had died. The memories of her provided incentive for a book for the general public (Moch, 1995). I dedicated the book to her.

Another woman with a great sense of humor asked that I present my research findings at her workplace. I agreed, and when we met, we had lunch, and I learned much more about her and her work. She was delighted with the reports of my research and was excited about the name I gave her in a book on breast cancer (Moch, 1995). She sent me a note and signed it the assigned name. In the note, she suggested that we meet again. We did meet again, and I learned even more about this woman whose humor made her so easy to be with. So how did my feelings of enjoying the company and the remarkable sense of humor this woman had affect my longitudinal study findings? I don't know.

Theoretical Underpinnings and Findings

How much does our own theoretical base affect the findings of research? Some qualitative perspectives and methods describe bracketing as a way of keeping theoretical perspectives in tow during the analysis phase of research. However, how capable of bracketing are researchers? For instance, I came to my research after years of practice with patients who had been diagnosed with a life-threatening illness and family support groups who were coping with a member who was seriously ill. I saw remarkable strengths in people dealing with the possibility of death. In my practice, I learned greatly from these people who were coping with life-threatening situations. I began my research with interest in knowing more about these families and was immediately attracted to crisis theory and Newman's theory of health as expanding consciousness (Newman, 1986, 1994). I know this interest and background affects my research, but how?

Knowing or Working With Research Participants

I conducted a pilot study on the experience of breast cancer with a convenience sample of midlife women in my community. Some of the people I interviewed were in my work environment, and some I saw frequently at various places in the community. It was difficult seeing the women and knowing whether or not to acknowledge them. I wondered whether I should tell them of the progress of the research or whether I should ask about their health. I also questioned what they thought when they saw me. Was I a reminder of their illness? Did they wonder whether I told others about their illness? Did they wish they hadn't had such intimate conversations with me?

This flood of questioning about research with people in my close environment made me wonder whether I would ever do another study so close to home. Having these feelings regularly when meeting these women in the community was and continues to be difficult. In future studies, I think I may try to find participants I would not regularly see. On the other hand, thinking such makes me wonder why. Do I feel I exploited these women? Do the women really feel what I think they feel? Maybe the women are happy to see me and through our encounter are reminded of their survivorship with cancer. One woman in another longitudinal study said she hoped I would see her in another 5 years and reinterview her again in the future as doing such would be a reminder that she was still alive. Maybe the women in my pilot study saw me in the same way that this woman saw me—as a comforting reminder about life.

What Is the Right Thing to Do?

The right thing to do as both a nurse and a researcher is not always clear. Many ethical questions emerge through health care research. Some of these questions will be discussed in Chapter 7. Often, the questions have to do with confidentiality and maintaining anonymity for the participant. Some questions have to do with whether or not to provide information to the participant that could be helpful for their health. Researchers struggle with these questions and sometimes discuss these issues with colleagues but rarely report their concerns in publications.

I struggled over whether I should write a book for the general public. When I talked to the participants, they encouraged me. They thought the book would be useful for encouraging family discussion. However, I wondered whether I could write about the women who had died. Who could give their permission?

I finally decided to get permission from family members. It was a difficult decision because maybe I was violating the confidentiality of my participants by doing so. One lady who had died, though, had been very excited about how the research interview had been helpful to her in discussing things with her husband. She had worried so much about finances and whether her husband wanted to spend so much on her treatment. She said, "What if we spend all this money, and I die anyway?" Between the first and second interview, she had discussed this with her husband. She reported the conversation during the second interview and felt happy about the outcome of the conversation with her husband. Because I knew she was influenced to discuss with her husband because of the interview, I thought she would have provided consent for the book.

Research Collaboration With Participants

I like to think of research participants as collaborators in research. I believe we jointly contribute to the evolution of knowledge. But, can we really be collaborators in the true sense of the word? I still have power over how the research is conducted and how the findings are presented. In Chapter 11, Krieger's (1991) and Behar's (1996) reflections shed light on this kind of questioning. They eloquently discuss their ideas in this regard. In my research with women diagnosed with breast cancer, I wanted to think of the women and the families as collaborators. When I have asked them to tell me whether or not I have captured the essence of their experience, they almost always agree. Maybe I have captured the essence, or maybe they don't feel comfortable disagreeing with me. I wonder if the participants feel comfortable "correcting" the researcher.

CONCLUSION

Many of the issues described will resurface in various ways throughout this book. Some of the authors will raise the same questions and share their reflections, much like I have done here. Some authors will also describe how they have resolved the issues. For instance, Gross, in the final chapter, describes her way of using the researcher experience to enhance her research. Her chapter, like some writings of the authors cited in Chapter 11, provides helpful guidance for dealing with the issues outlined for the researcher experience in health care research. In addition, Chapter 3, "Sensitive Issues in Life Story Research," Chapter 7,

"Processing the Researcher Experience Through Discussion," and Chapter 9, "Qualitative Researchers Working as Teams," provide suggestions for dealing with some of the issues.

REFERENCES

Behar, R. (1996). *The vulnerable observer: Anthropology that breaks your heart.* Boston: Beacon.

Krieger, S. (1991). *Social science and the self.* New Brunswick, NJ: Rutgers University Press.

Moch, S. D. (1990). Health within the experience of breast cancer. *Journal of Advanced Nursing, 15,* 1426-1435.

Moch, S. D. (1995). *Breast cancer: Twenty women's stories.* New York: National League for Nursing Press.

Moch, S. D. (1998). Health within illness: Concept development through research and practice. *Journal of Advanced Nursing, 28,* 305-310.

Newman, M. A. (1986). *Health as expanding consciousness.* St. Louis: C. V. Mosby.

Newman, M. A. (1994). *Health as expanding consciousness* (2nd ed.). New York: National League for Nursing Press.

3

Sensitive Issues in Life Story Research

Sheila K. Smith

In many realms of contemporary life, intimate stories on sensitive issues have become commonplace. Narratives of personal distress and adversity are encountered in many settings and seem to serve both personal and wider social purposes. Plummer (1995), for instance, describes the latter part of the 20th century as "cluttered" with problematic sexual stories. Widespread and previously unheard tales of difficult sex-gender experiences have proliferated in therapy groups, book circuits, TV talk shows, and in the news media. In research as well, entry into personal, sensitive topics has gained greater acceptance—partly because of human studies' efforts to more fully understand the complexities of human subjectivity and agency, but also as part of an expanding social dialogue in which previously invisible or politically marginalized voices are now claiming credibility as part of the normative human center. Feminist and critical social research approaches, in particular, have expedited the process of telling sensitive human stories as research.

Personal story told as research is still new enough to evoke powerful transformations among its audiences. For example, in my own research on women's experiences of victimizing sexualization (Smith, 1996, 1997a, 1997b), the participants, myself as researcher, academic colleagues, and multiple listening audiences have described experiences ranging from personal validation to altered social understandings to changed identity configurations in response to meanings articulated through the research. The act of constructing a life story, whether as actively engaged in by the one constructing the story or as secondarily engaged in by an engaged listener, has a powerful, potentially transforming, (re)organizational impact.

The outcome of telling a story is never clear in advance, however, and an opposing potential is present as well: the potential to disempower, degrade, or pathologize, whether through simple exposure, failure of response, or distortions through objectification. Researchers who use narrative approaches to investigate sensitive topics sometimes walk a fine line between these opposing outcomes. This chapter will explore these and other issues in describing aspects of the researcher experience with highly personal, sensitive issues.

THEORETICAL PERSPECTIVES

Life story, or personal narrative, has been used in nursing research to gain access to personal and wider social meanings associated with some of the more difficult and sensitive issues in health and human caring. Giving voice to the subject by eliciting, interpreting, and presenting narratives of human health experience has contributed to understanding those experiences, as well as to understanding how people make sense of their lived social world. Studying human health as an interpretive process of studying meanings has been part of what has been described as the *paradigm of pattern* (Newman, 1994) in nursing. Pattern, or the life course developmental progression of person-environment interaction, can be identified and made accessible as a coherent expression of life structure and subjective experience of self-in-the-world. Through researcher-participant collaboration in the process of narrative inquiry, meanings, events, and experiences are made mutually comprehensible, resulting in the development of new points of access for acting in the world (Smith, 1996). Narrative approaches are thus an important mechanism for the construction of agency. They can therefore be used for both research and practice, and extensive multidisciplinary literature supports their use for both purposes.

Life story methodologies may be particularly well suited to understanding and integrating adverse life experiences. The manner in which adversity is understood and managed over time has been described by Cohler (1991) and Antonovsky (1987) as requiring the maintenance of a coherent life story. The capacity to maintain narrative coherence has been proposed to include complex portrayals of self and others, emphasizing the reflexive quality of subjective understanding. Perhaps especially for life circumstances experienced as unanticipated or beyond personal control, the ability to organize a convincing explanatory framework, and assign meaning to otherwise incomprehensible events, may be key to processes of restoring agentic engagement with one's personal and social worlds. Narrative and patterning theories suggest that such developments are relational in nature. The ability to discern uniquely patterned events and experiences, as well as to manage personal versus cultural meanings, may be facilitated through the reflexive process of engagement and connection in telling one's personal story. In telling the life story, the exceptional and the ordinary are seen side by side. Points of connection are discerned so that the exceptional becomes integrated or understood as a coherent and meaningful aspect of personal history.

TAKING THE SOCIAL TURN

Women's' agentic development in particular has been shown to be facilitated by accurately locating one's self in the world (Haraway, 1988; Harding, 1989). By becoming cognizant of one's unique personal history and adversity as reflections of broader social relations, access to a less personalized interpretive stance is afforded. Women's developmental research now suggests that less personalized understanding of sex/gender experience may be important for developing resistance to objectification and disempowerment (Rogers, 1991).

Narrative approaches have been central to feminist interpretive research, both in terms of deconstructing cultural beliefs about women and generating new knowledge about women's lives. Personal narrative simultaneously uses and generates women's life stories as primary research documents (Personal Narratives Group, 1989). Personal narratives "illuminate the course of a life over time and allows for its interpretation in its historical and cultural context" (p. 4). The research process of "giving form to a whole life" (p. 4) requires that the researcher engage in interpretive acts, considering the meaning of individual and social dynamics. Narratives recount personal processes of constructing self and reveal the dynamic interactions between individual agency, consciousness, and social structure, thereby providing descriptions of social life from a specific vantage point (Anderson, Armitage, Jack, & Wittner, 1990). Because such a vantage point often reveals invisible and neglected areas of experience, the process of interpreting women's lives allows understandings of gender dynamics to emerge at both individual and social-system levels (Personal Narratives Group, 1989). By engaging in this process, women are able to provide depictions of how they understand themselves within their worlds, how they understand "the social relationships and institutions that [make up] the worlds they [live] in and how they [act] to preserve or restructure those relationships" (Anderson et al., 1990, p. 106).

USE OF NARRATIVE IN RESARCH AND PRACTICE

As can be seen, we are in a time of particular interest in personal narrative. Expressions of uncertainty and disorganized meaning, within the individual and within wider social bounds, are poorly tolerated by many. The ability to tell a life story that can be understood by self and by others has been shown to facilitate meaning-making, integrity, and personal coherence. Contemplating one's life, making it whole and comprehensible, are often equated with seeking value and purpose, political consciencization, achieving balance and health, or spiritual transformation. A cautionary note must be sounded, however. Pattern recognition and narrative integrity can be difficult accomplishments. Significant time, skill, and empathic connection are required for the remaking of self and agentic reinterpretation described here as research and practice. The potential for personal world disruption is very real, as events and experiences previously construed as separate and disconnected, but laden with personal distress, are reinterpreted as part of a larger explanatory framework. In our tell-all world, significant vulnerability may attend an overly simplified or inadequately conceptualized approach to working with life stories.

My own research used a qualitative, interpretive method to elicit major themes and patterns of women's experiences of victimizing sexualization and healing (Smith, 1996, 1997a, 1997b). The focus of the research was participants' lived experiences of growing up female and sexual, for women who self-identified their sex-gender experiences as having been harmful to them. The research combined feminist social epistemologies with nursing's health patterning framework (Newman, 1994) to identify composite effects of sex-gender harm over the course of a lifetime. Concepts of self, subjectivity, relational growth, and developmental change were emphasized. At the center of these life stories, however, were experiences of suffering, loss, betrayal, and powerlessness—dynamics of disintegration that required virtually these women's entire adult lives to reconcile. Overall, victimizing sexualization was described as a long-term, substantive experience of loss and violation of one's relational and sexual self. Healing experiences were characterized as long and difficult processes of self- and relational transformation (Smith, 1996).

Applying the questions and methods of feminist inquiry to the nursing concerns of health and human caring inevitably led to a research project involving highly personal and sensitive subject matter, on several levels. Most evident and perhaps easiest to anticipate was the sensitive nature of the topic itself: the complexities of harmful sex-gender experiences and their personal, family, relational, and community-cultural convolutions. By looking for patterns in these experiences (i.e., meaningful explanations of ways the experiences hung together), the project required attending to interconnections on all these levels. This included finding the *content* connections between sex-gender harm and health patterning in the interview data, as well as the *political* connections of personal harm, disempowerment, and gender inequalities. In ways that were less easily anticipated, it also included experiential and epistemologic connections between myself as researcher and the women whose lives I was entering into; and transforming personal connections among those of us who shared in the obscurities of creating theory from various health patterning research projects. The sensitive nature of the research topic was reflected at all four of these levels, with implications for the researcher experience at each.

CONTENT CONNECTIONS

Sensitive issues of content emerged early in the research and continued throughout the study. Candidates for the study were self-identified based on circulated criteria; all had experienced sexual and relational abuse. The severity of the abuse, number of occurrences, time span over which the abuse occurred, and perpetrators of the abuse varied widely. Participants' degree of developmental movement through healing and reconciliation processes varied widely as well, with two participants still clearly experiencing considerable trauma from their experiences.

Two others were dropped from the study early on, as they were deemed not stable enough to participate. Both women were unable to remain focused on the content of the study, evidenced awkward and less than fully open interaction dynamics, and did not follow through with planned research meetings. From the perspective available at the conclusion of the study, these behaviors may have been evidence of some of the very patterning configurations through which it would be most beneficial to engage with clients in practice relationships.

Because of the high level of abuse represented in participants' experiences, I was extremely careful with all participants to assess for their reactions to the research throughout the study. The women's reactions were used as a guide for proceeding or not proceeding with specific discussions and for scheduling follow-up appointments. I spoke directly with each participant about the potential for increased distress in telling their experiences and emphasized the need to avoid any retraumatizing through their research involvement. Four participants were asked to consult with their mental health providers prior to participating in the study. They did this, and mutual decisions were made regarding their continuation in the study. Participants expressed a wide array of feelings and responses during their research involvement.

The narrative process of telling their experiences was difficult for several of the women. Some were missing memories, had difficulty thinking clearly, and jumbled the historical sequencing of their experiences. Unclear and vague references sometimes required long periods of listening to discern correct ordering and relational connections. Widely varying levels of emotional connection with their experiences were revealed. Several women went through periods of emotional distress during the interviews, demonstrated by increased disorganization of their thoughts, unsteady voices, physically shaking and getting cold, increased nervous activity, becoming silent, increased speed of cognitive associations, and descriptions of memory flooding and visual flashbacks.

Through all of this, however, it was apparent that all participants were trying hard to convey an organized sense of their experiences. For three women, the ending place of the research was clearly painful. New memories and insights had developed that were uncomfortable and unsettling. Even so, these women felt they had made important progress and were not unhappy with their involvement in the study. All three indicated they felt better about themselves and were more assured about the validity and meaning of their experiences.

Some participants experienced increased distress during the research because of other ongoing life events. Participants were engaged in new therapy work, difficult legal proceedings, exacerbations of other health problems, medication changes, an additional assault experience, new relationships, and external confirmation of memories that had surfaced prior to the start of the research, to name a few. All of these women chose to remain in the study and felt they had the professional support they needed to manage their experiences. The possibility that the research interviewing interacted with other life difficulties cannot be discounted, however, and emphasizes the need for researchers to be adequately prepared for assessing, supporting, responding, referring, and making sound decisions about continued research involvement.

POLITICAL CONNECTIONS

Data from this study support the feminist perspective that victimizing sexualization can operate as a dimension of health patterning through broader social spheres of young women's lives. Because of the social and political complexities of sex-gender relationships, several participants did not fully understand the focus of the study at the beginning of the research. This was especially true for components related to social relations of gender, social meanings about women's sexuality, and broader social patterns of women's subordination. This limited how much interpretive content some participants could include about their experiences but did not exclude examples of these levels from emerging in their stories. Socially constructed gender-related and sexuality-related power imbalances were discernable in heterosexual, family, and community dynamics. Home and family environments were frequently described as reflecting the control and subordination of power-structured gender relations. Examples of negative community attitudes toward girls and women, gender-based double standards of behavior, and discriminatory treatment were identified by virtually every participant. In some cases, perceptions of community-wide scapegoating and devaluing of women were expressed, interacting as well with examples of racial and religious intolerance. By becoming cognizant of the sex-gender dynamics that characterized their personal relational development, several participants also became aware of these broader political aspects of women's social positions. Some of the women rejected these understandings, whereas others embraced them, providing these women with powerful and less personalized explanations for their individual difficulties and with focal points for an emerging or evolving sense of agency and social justice. Several participants expressed a need for stronger understandings of the social world, feeling they would have been much better able to protect themselves from relational violations and unwanted sexual experiences if they'd understood that these were characteristics of the culture, rather than faults or deficits within themselves.

RESEARCHER-PARTICIPANT CONNECTIONS

The narrative process resulted in substantive personal changes for both the investigator and participants. Participants were seen to develop new insights into their personal experiences, family relationships, and social world understandings. They declared stronger feelings of self-value and personal rights; expressed increased confidence in the validity of their own perceptions; experienced greater integration of past events into their present sense of self; and presented an overall more centered, grounded, and self-cohering demeanor. My involvement as investigator resulted in a significant increase in my own understandings of abuse dynamics and the complexities of growth processes. Hearing the women's information was at first painful and anxiety provoking. I was aware of attempts to protect the participants from their own pain and distress. Over time, these worries diminished, and I experienced a sense of growing with the participants. My appreciation for the complexity of the human condition grew considerably as each woman moved along in her ability to formulate an increasingly accessible depiction of her life, resulting in a deeply felt sense of understanding and connection with virtually all of the women in the study.

COLLEGIAL CONNECTIONS

The last way in which this research facilitated connections was among a group of research colleagues, all of whom were immersed in health patterning research as dissertation students. Led by our adviser, Dr. Margaret Newman (1994), we met regularly to discuss our findings and respond to each other's work. Our interactive process of thought and analysis resulted not only in clarifications for each of us as individuals but in extensions and clarifications of health patterning theory itself. One student (Lamendola, 1998) was able to describe aspects of caring and connection that lead to personal gratification among highly committed expert nurses in palliative care. Merian Litchfield (1997) described the process of nurse-family transitions in health patterning as she worked within research relationships with families experiencing complex health concerns. My own research (Smith, 1996) contributed understandings of ways in which the lived social world simultaneously shapes and is reflected within an individual's health patterning configurations over time, opening the way for using health patterning as a framework for additional health research into substantive social concerns. Endo (1996) was able to explain the relational process of pattern recognition as a developmental intervention with cancer patients. Tommet (1997) described family crises and aspects of development that occurred through the experiences of raising a child with very fragile health. Our work together surely catalyzed each of us to greater accomplishments than we would ever have managed on our own and provided a very important avenue for managing and integrating our own growth and change as it evolved through our narrative connections with those whose lives we sought to understand. This activity was an excellent example of ways in which dialogue and narrative inquiry function to produce and organize knowledge. We became agents of knowledge in an interactive process, opening new opportunities for ourselves and others to act in the world. Through interaction and dialogue, we developed shared examples of some of the ways in which the production of knowledge is indeed an integrative social practice. Because of the substantive way that activities such as these shape the directions and paradigms of an evolving discipline, careful attention is required to the social and epistemic consequences of the resulting knowledge.

These aspects of the researcher experience with sensitive issues in life story research demonstrate ways in which narrative inquiry and health patterning research operate at many levels to produce new knowledge and exert significant personal and social impact. Of particular interest to me is the applicability of concepts and understandings from feminist social constructionism to these observations (Hartman & Messer-Davidow, 1991): By emphasizing both agent-initiated and system-imposed change or resistance to change, the practices of "knowers" become potentially powerful practices of individual and social change.

REFERENCES

Anderson, K., Armitage, S., Jack, D., & Wittner, J. (1990). Beginning where we are: Feminist methodology in oral history. In J. M. Nielson (Ed.), *Feminist research methods.* Boulder: Westview.

Antonovsky, A. (1987). *Unraveling the mystery of health: How people manage stress and stay well.* San Francisco: Jossey-Bass.

Cohler, B. J. (1991). The life story and the study of resilience and response to adversity. *Journal of Narrative and Life History, 1*(2&3), 169-200.

Endo, E. (1996). *Pattern recognition as a nursing intervention with adults with cancer.* Unpublished doctoral dissertation, University of Minnesota, Minneapolis.

Haraway, D. (1988). Situated knowledges: The science question in feminism and the privilege of partial perspective. *Feminist Studies, 14*(3), 575-599.

Harding, S. (Ed.). (1989). *Feminism and methodology.* Bloomington: Indiana University Press.

Hartman, J. E., & Messer-Davidow, E. (Eds.). (1991). *(En)Gendering knowledge: Feminists in Academe.* Knoxville: University of Tennessee Press.

Lamendola, F. (1998). *Patterns of the caregiving experiences of selected nurses in hospice and HIV/AIDS care.* Unpublished doctoral dissertation, University of Minnesota, Minneapolis.

Litchfield, M. (1997). *The process of nursing partnerships in family health.* Unpublished doctoral dissertation, University of Minnesota, Minneapolis.

Newman, M. A. (1994). *Health as expanding consciousness* (2nd ed.). New York: National League for Nursing.

Personal Narratives Group. (Ed.). (1989). *Interpreting women's lives: Feminist theory and personal narratives.* Bloomington: Indiana University Press.

Plummer, K. (1995). *Telling sexual stories: Power, change and social worlds.* London: Routledge.

Rogers, A. G. (1991). A feminist poetics of psychotherapy. In C. Gilligan, A. G. Rogers, & D. L. Tolman (Eds.), *Women, girls and psychotherapy: Reframing resistance.* New York: Haworth.

Smith, S. K. (1996). *Women's experiences of victimizing sexualization and healing.* Unpublished doctoral dissertation, University of Minnesota, Minneapolis.

Smith, S. K. (1997a). Women's experiences of victimizing sexualization: Part I. Responses related to abuse and home and family environment. *Issues in Mental Health Nursing, 18,* 395-416.

Smith, S. K. (1997b). Women's experiences of victimizing sexualization: Part II. Community and longer term personal impacts. *Issues in Mental Health Nursing, 18,* 417-432.

Tommet, P. (1997). *Nurse-parent dialogue: Illuminating the pattern of families with children who are medically fragile.* Unpublished doctoral dissertation, University of Minnesota, Minneapolis.

4

The Researcher Experience in Health Care Research With Families

Marie F. Gates

Nancy R. Lackey

Using qualitative research designs in conducting research with families is a recently valued phenomenon. Researchers in the areas of nursing, social sciences, education, women's studies, and family therapy (Handel, 1992; LaRossa & Wolf, 1985; Rosenblatt & Fischer, 1993; Uphold & Strickland, 1989; Whall & Fawcett, 1991) have identified the need to explore a variety of research designs, analyses, and results that will accurately represent problems and concerns reflected by families. Deatrick, Faux, and Moore (1993), in their review of articles on the experience of families dealing with a child with chronic illness, found 100 qualitative studies on the topic. Published reports of the researcher experiences while doing family qualitative studies have not been so common (Gubrium & Holstein, 1991, 1993; LaRossa & Wolf, 1985). A recent exception has been the weaving of experiences in an excellent text on qualitative methods in family research (Gilgun, Daly, & Handel, 1992). Focus on the research experience itself has gained more attention over the past few years at qualitative research conferences, in part due to increased focus on feminist and critical social theory methods in qualitative research (Campbell & Bunting, 1991). The thesis of this book assumes that there is a need to better understand what issues surround the steps of qualitative research regarding families. The purpose of this chapter is to highlight those perplexing events or issues, based on researcher experience, that frequently occur in designing and conducting qualitative studies with families. Examples from the literature are provided, along with personal illustrations and concerns related to the researcher experience.

This chapter is organized according to major steps of the research process. The following issues are included in this discussion: defining family, deciding and stating the problem and research question(s), identifying an appropriate qualitative design or a combination of designs, sampling, selecting methods of collecting data, conducting data analysis, interpreting the results, and investigating ethical issues that are specific to family research. These steps are not necessarily linear. For organizational convenience, the steps are listed as proceeding consecutively, as one would prepare a proposal or manuscript; however, previous steps may be revisited, which frequently happens in real qualitative family research.

ISSUES REGARDING DEFINITIONS OF *FAMILY*

One of the first issues that the researcher has to deal with is how to identify who constitutes the family. Conducting qualitative research involves studying families as they are, in context. To do this, the concept of family has to be defined. In our experience, this is probably one of the hardest decisions that must be made. Discussion of who family is starts early in the conceptualization phase and recurs as the study progresses.

In 1979, Burr, Hill, Nye, and Reiss wrote that sociologists did not need to define family because their audiences already knew what the term meant—a nuclear family—father, mother, and children. In our mobile society of today, family structure can take many forms other than the nuclear family—single-parent families with children; grandparents with grandchildren; gay and lesbian couples with or without children; extended families; families composed of surrogate aunts, uncles, and grandparents. Some families even count neighbors, close friends, church members, and pets as part of their family. Gubrium and Holstein (1991) suggest that only families know who their members are. A family is not so much a concrete set of social ties as a way of attaching meaning to interpersonal relations.

The difficulty of defining the concept of family has been explored ad infinitum. Definitions have been put forth by sociologists, psychologists, anthropologists, and lawyers, but no one term fits all (Johnson, 1998). Therefore, the consensus of researchers is that the definition of family is what the family says it is. The following example illustrates the complexity that one researcher had in determining who should be considered members of a specific family. Malone (1997) intended to study how families adjusted to the problems of a son who had either a mental illness or chronic disease. Her initial definition of family consisted of the parents and children living together in the same environment. Soon after Malone started her data collection, she realized she needed to include the Bishop of the Mormon Ward in her definition of family. Therefore, in her study, several interviews with families needed to include the Bishop (J. Malone, personal communication, July 23, 1998).

The issue of defining family affects all steps of the qualitative research process, such as selecting who to sample from the family, determining the unit of analysis, interpreting the results, and deciding which family member(s) would verify these results. The issue of defining family alone may dissuade researchers from attempting family research in general and qualitative family research in particular. Should the researcher have a set definition for family, which may restrict the nature of the research? Or should the researcher use the broad, more flexible definition that family members are whoever the family says they are? Although we as researchers can intellectually accept the definition of family as whoever the family says they are, we are concerned about whether reviewers of grant proposals or manuscript editors will agree with this definition when the number of members in family dwindles to only two.

ISSUES REGARDING STATEMENT OF
THE PROBLEM AND RESEARCH QUESTION(S)

The first step of the process is deciding what the problem is and how the research question(s) should be stated. The decisions made in this step, along with the definition of family and type of family research, will ultimately determine the qualitative design, sample, procedure, and analysis of the results of the proposed study.

Feetham (1991) identifies two major types of family research: *family-related research* and *family research*. Family-related research refers to research that focuses on nonlinear relationships between family members. This type of research calls for description, explanation, or prediction about the family, based on data typically collected from individual family members. In contrast, family research calls for collection of data focusing on the family as a whole. Of the two methods, family research is the most complex and the most difficult to conceptualize and execute. A program of research that includes both types can add depth and breadth to the knowledge of the family.

While conceptualizing the research problem and question(s), the researcher needs to decide, using the selected definition, whether he or she will be using the family-related or family research method. Once this decision is made, then the researcher will know how to write the research question(s). If the family-related research method is selected, the researcher will develop question(s) that individual members can respond to and relate the answer to their family. Selecting family research method will involve developing question(s) that elicit data from the family as a whole in terms of structure or function. (Feetham, 1991).

Along with Feetham's (1991) description of family research, Gilgun's (1992) comments help shape the description of qualitative family research. Gilgun describes qualitative family research as

> research with a focus on experiences within families as well as between families and outside systems; data are words or pictures and not numbers; the data are conceptualized, collected, analyzed, and interpreted qualitatively; the subjects or informants of the research are persons who mutually define themselves as family, are in committed relationships, have a shared sense of personal history, and who usually but not always have legal and biological ties. (p. 24)

Here, we will share our experience in attempting an ill-fated family needs study. It was part of a larger study (Lackey & Gates, 1994), which also explored patient and caregiver needs (Gates, Lackey, & White, 1995; Harrington, Lackey, & Gates, 1996). We will discuss the family part of the study here and again later in the chapter. The purpose of the family part of the study was to determine the needs of the family when one member within that family had cancer and was receiving services from either a cancer clinic or a hospice. In attempting to formulate the question for the study, we decided we wanted to compare family needs as identified by family members individually (family-related research) and by the family as a whole (family research). We also thought the study met Gilgun's (1992) requirement for defining qualitative family research: it dealt with the experiences of the family, it was relevant to the family as they saw themselves as family, the data would be provided in the form of words, and it would include as many of the family who wished to or could participate. (We never published the results of this portion of our study because we never attained large enough numbers to warrant publishing it as a research-based article. We periodically debated how we could publish our experiences as an issues-based article. This chapter provided us with an opportunity to refer to our process and experience in this study.)

ISSUES OF QUALITATIVE DESIGN

Which qualitative design is best for studying families? Is a single methodology better than a combination of designs? The design in both family-related and family research needs to be congruent with the problem statement or question(s). Phenomenology and ethnomethodology are the major kinds of methods used in qualitative family research (Gubrium & Holstein, 1993). Gilgun (1992) further suggests a variety of other methods and combinations of methods that include critical social theory, feminist theory, and so on. No one qualitative approach is deemed the most appropriate for family qualitative research (Rosen-blatt & Fischer, 1993).

In the family needs study mentioned earlier (Lackey & Gates, 1994), we chose naturalistic inquiry as the design of choice. For another study, looking at the experiences, life ways, and needs of youngsters under the age of 18 caring for adults with cancer in the home (Gates & Lackey, 1998), we selected three quali-tative approaches: phenomenology, ethnography, and unstructured survey. We chose these approaches because we were studying a phenomenon that had not been extensively described. The three approaches provided more breadth and depth in understanding the phenomenon. Each of us collected data related to our method of expertise; for example, Lackey is more proficient in phenomenology and Gates in ethnography.

SAMPLING ISSUES

A qualitative study typically includes a nonprobability type of sample, such as network or purposive. Thomas (1987) suggests there is an innate bias in recruit-ing and selecting families for qualitative research. Using the example of her qualitative study with families caring for children who are ventilator dependent, Thomas identifies region of the country, types of parents, and whether physi-cians will provide names of families for selection as examples of ways her own study had limits placed on which families might even be considered, let alone se-lected, for a qualitative study.

Once families are identified, will they then agree to be in the study and will they agree to include all or only some of their members, regardless of how they define family? One needs at least two members to make a family unit. How many should there be in a qualitative study? Moriarty & Cotroneo (1993) discuss in-clusion criteria for quantitative family studies and suggest two and usually three as the typical family configurations that are sampled. Again two or three tends to be what is reported in qualitative literature. But how many members really are enough to constitute a family?

Going back to our experience with the ill-fated family needs study (Lackey & Gates, 1994), we found the logistics for obtaining sufficient numbers of families posed problems for us and led to our failure to have a large enough sample of families. We asked the person with cancer to identify who he or she saw as fam-ily. Although the person could and would identify who was family, there was re-luctance in providing names beyond the primary caregiver. One reason often ex-pressed by patients was that they did not wish to impose an additional burden on their family members who were already doing other things for them. If the per-son with cancer was willing to give us names, identified family members might refuse because they either did not have time or did not believe they had needs. Giving away any precious time to another project, no matter how worthwhile, was not a priority. Some patients did not have other family members living in the area. This ill-fated study was conducted in a large Southern city. Despite the stereotype of large, extended Southern families, many patients did not have family members living near them, as they were scattered around the country and the world. Family conflicts often precluded the patient from including all members who were really part of the family. So how many families did we finally obtain? Of 69 potential families recruited for the total study, (Lackey & Gates, 1994) six families in clinic settings agreed to do individual family member surveys, with two of those families also doing so as a group; in hospice settings, 11 families provided data as individual family members, only three of those as a family group. Numbers within the families themselves ranged from two to five. Getting families together took time and energy. We are not sure whether we would have had the stamina to gather all 69 family groups.

ISSUES IN COLLECTING DATA

Examples of problems and issues related to the researcher experience in collecting data were more prevalent in the literature than were issues related to other aspects of the qualitative process. Interviewing tended to be the predominant form of data collection. Interviews involved individual family members, dyads, or larger groups (or a combination of these). Individual or dyad interviews were more common. Where both individual and larger family interviews took place, differences in data tended to occur. For example, Thomas (1987) found differences provided by individual and groups in her ventilator-dependent study. In each of the families, reports of individual data differed from family data in such areas as family secrets shared and assessments of other member's strengths and weaknesses.

Astedt-Kurki (1996) also reported about the trials and tribulations of conducting family group interviews in her study on how families viewed their health as a family. She, too, found families needed to convey harmony or were reluctant to identify opposing views. She, too, wondered whether young children can really be involved. If the subject is too abstract or difficult, they may not be able to contribute. Astedt-Kurki reported that adolescents found it difficult to concentrate or thought the subject was not important. In that situation, Astedt-Kurki suggested the possibility of separate interviews for the children. She also found that the families continued to talk about the situation between interviews. Often, they came to interesting conclusions without the interviewer being present. She saw the family interviews as dialogues between and among family members who were present. She also reported that family members' talking together between interviews served as a way of coming to terms regarding what the experience meant to them—often in a positive manner.

Gates (1994), in conducting interviews of couples who had experienced a hysterectomy, also found that both the woman and her partner engaged in dialogue about the experience, often taking turns, less frequently talking together, and coming to consensus about the experience and what it meant to them. They engaged in such dialogue during the interviews and between interviews, as well.

Rosenblatt and Fischer (1993) spoke to other methods of collecting data, such as observation and use of diaries and letters. Observation can take place in person, through field observation, or with cameras and video, as Murphy (1992) did in her study of sibling-infant relationships. Murphy reinforced the need to use more than one technique in collecting data, for example, interviewing parents, observing children and infants, and using drawings.

On the other hand, LaRossa, Bennett, and Gelles (1981) say qualitative family researchers tend to rely more heavily on interviewing, because the intimacy and privacy of family may preclude prolonged observation. In studying nine families, Murphy (1992) observed all members of the family for 1 year. In that time, she was able to observe parenting strategies, parental variation of interest in their children, pattern variations over time and day. Although she did not speculate on the effects of her experience of conducting this type of study, one can wonder about such questions as, What it was like being there with the families during meal or bath times? Did she consider her presence an intrusion? Did the families? How did her presence affect the data?

When Gates spent time with families in the study of adolescent and child caregivers of adults with cancer (Gates & Lackey, 1998), she went to schools and outings with the children and was around the family during dinner times and caregiving times. Did she feel out or place? No. Did she wonder if her presence affected the care of the family member? Perhaps. The children seemed to do what came naturally to them. Based on her experiences with children and adolescents over time, she did not think the events that she observed were affected by her presence. But who knows?

Handel (1992) talked about the importance of using children in families when conducting family-related or family research. The age of the child and the ability of the child to understand the questions being studied become critical here. At what age can children be involved? For example, while conducting the phenomenology interviews for the young caregiver study (Gates & Lackey, 1998), Lackey found children aged 8 to 12 required many prompts to elicit their experiences and feelings regarding caring for a family member with cancer. She concluded that a variety of questions and prompts to stimulate the children's responses were more appropriate than a broad overall question in soliciting the feelings and experiences for this age group. Walsh (1998) and Yarrow (1960) concurred with the use of multiple strategies for eliciting data.

When children are in the home and are willing to be included in data collection, it might be helpful to obtain data from various configurations of family

When children are in the home and are willing to be included in data collection, it might be helpful to obtain data from various configurations of family members at the same time. Cromwell and Peterson (1981) suggested that the multisystem-multitrait paradigm in which data is collected from individuals, dyads, and the family as a whole be used more often in studying families. We would like to incorporate that technique in studying families where a child or adolescent is providing care to an adult with a chronic physical illness. Using the multi- system-multitrait paradigm for collecting data from the youngster, the person with the illness, and the parent, both alone and in groups, would provide more helpful data than individual interviews alone.

As we reviewed the way we collected our data in the ill-fated family needs study (Lackey & Gates, 1994), we discovered that we had used the same question for the identification of needs for both individual family members and for families as a group: "What are my needs as a family member of a patient with cancer?" We were surprised that we obtained different data. The process we used in collecting the data from the individual members was to provide them with the survey and ask them to fill it out. For the family groups, we asked them to fill out the survey as a group. One of us was present during both the individual and group data collection. In retrospect, we should have worded the question differently for the family considering the question as a group.

ISSUES REGARDING
DATA ANALYSIS

In discussing qualitative data analysis, Rosenblatt and Fischer (1993) highlighted the importance of specifying the analytic method used. For example, if the study is phenomenological, what specific phenomenological analysis was used? If a specific analysis was selected for the proposal yet the data collected did not yield itself to this analysis method, could the analysis method be changed without violating the assumptions? Deciding what to code and how to code is important. If data are obtained from varying family system levels, will they be analyzed together, separately, or both? What happens if differences are found in individual data and group data? Which data will be reported (Rosenblatt & Fischer, 1993)? Gilgun (1992) believes you need multiple forms of data. Data analysis, then, would require line-by-line investigation of written material, review of videotapes, and decisions regarding ways to look for interaction strategies.

Returning to our ill-fated family needs example (Lackey & Gates, 1994), the individual answers gave us 145 different items, which could serve as a basis for a family questionnaire or survey. Data from individual family members referred to such examples: "Basically, I don't have many needs, I am more concerned

Whereas the group answers tended to be broad, consensus answers related to the patient, such as "doing for her whatever she wants"; or family togetherness needs, such as "pulling together," or "we need to know the full extent of the treatment in order to be the most helpful and supportive we can be to attend to the patient's needs"; or family financial needs—such as "money to get what we need for her and for us"; or abstract terms, such as "cooperation," "love," or "patience."

We had hoped to identify family need items. We found that the families, when meeting together, persuaded each other to go along with the more global items. Individual differences were not attended to. Capturing both perspectives provided both individual need items and family consensus items. We did not have a large enough sample of families to do further analysis, interpretation, or instrument development, which had been our original purpose.

ISSUES IN INTERPRETING THE RESULTS

While interpreting the results of a qualitative study, the qualitative researcher constantly wonders about getting the "truth." Is the family giving researchers the truth, information that they think researchers want to hear, or how they want to portray themselves in society (Gubrium & Holsten, 1993; Rosenblatt & Fischer, 1993)? When interpreting family data, family and individual developmental theories, family theories, systems theories, and culture theories all play a role. How many of these theories do we incorporate and refer to as we interpret the data and come to our conclusions? Families are complex; can those complexities be truly accounted for?

ETHICAL ISSUES

Several ethical issues pertinent in family qualitative research were found in the literature. For example, Demi and Warren (1995) speak to the ethical concern of subjective interpretation. Because qualitative data are analyzed for meaning, researchers may impose their own logic and values on what is communicated by the family. Researchers may change the data collection process and ask questions of more than one member if the individual targeted does not provide the data needed. Regarding ethical issues, what happens when all family members do not want to participate? In that instance, can the researcher really say that an individual speaks for the family as a whole?

Another issue relates to obtaining consent. When you are seeking family permission, is it best to have all family members together and obtain full and complete consents, or is it better to explain the study to one member of the family and hope that correct information is conveyed to others? Astedt-Kurki (1996) reported a situation in her study on family experiences and well-being that speaks to the need for getting truly informed consent from each individual family member. She discussed consent and the data collection process only with the mother and found some reluctance on the father's part because he was unaware that the interview would be tape-recorded.

Are children's decisions to participate really their decisions? It is considered important to obtain the assent of children (Berry, Dodd, Hinds, & Ferrell, 1996; Consensus Conference on Guidelines for Adolescent Health Research, 1995). Do children truly give their own assent or do they agree to participate because of their need for attention, coercion by parents, or research incentives?

On the other hand, when children under the age of 18 are part of the family, a parent may just assume the child would not wish to participate without asking the child. For example, in the study of young caregivers (Gates & Lackey, 1998), one 14-year-old had responsibility for the care of her mother with breast cancer. The mother was approached about her daughter's participation and refused to give consent. The mother informed her daughter about the study and explained that she did not give permission, thinking the daughter would not want to be involved. The daughter became extremely upset—saying she had "a lot to say" and was especially concerned that her mother would not let her have input in the decision regarding participation. As a result, the mother called the next morning and reversed her decision.

LaRossa and colleagues (1981) talked about flexible design as contributing to difficulty with informed consent. How can you tell a potential participant about the questions when you may change them during data collection? Because family is so pervasive for most people, the researcher may not be able to specify everything that may be covered in the study. Because, too, qualitative family research relies so heavily on interviews, the researcher could assume a cross-examining attitude and thus place constraints on individual or group family. In conjoint interviewing, people may not really want to answer a question but feel coerced to do so if another person answers the question. The ambience of the home setting, such as meeting over coffee or at the kitchen table, may suggest that "you're among friends," so family members may say more than they mean or wish to. Unexpected phone calls or the appearance of visitors may inadvertently become part of the study. These situations contribute to a more overriding ethical burden that occurs for the researcher who is doing qualitative family research.

Writers have spoken to the issue of family qualitative research being mistaken for therapy. Thomas (1987) compared research interviews with therapeutic interviews and found they were often similar. However, in research interviews, the intent is not focused on changing the person or family involved nor on providing therapy. Daly (1992) suggests that to counteract such a mistaken assumption on the family's part, the nature of the research be explained explicitly. Then, the families are not as likely to approach the session as a therapeutic one, even though it may turn out to be so.

Moriarity and Cotroneo (1993) provided a helpful summary on ethical issues that are critical for researchers engaged in qualitative family research. Areas qualitative researchers need to reflect on include: obtaining multiple consent, assent and consent of any children involved, avoiding even subtle coercion, making sure all participants involved comprehend the risks and benefits, protecting voluntariness, and suggesting options to family if an issue is sensitive or affect laden.

We have raised questions, provided few answers. We have attempted to stimulate discussion related to the effects of the researcher experience through phases of conducting qualitative family research. As we conclude this chapter, we found more illustrations woven into reports of studies than we thought existed. More are needed.

REFERENCES

Astedt-Kurki, P. (1996). The family interview: Exploring experiences of family health and well-being. *Journal of Advanced Nursing, 24,* 506-511.

Berry, D., Dodd, M., Hinds, P. S., & Ferrell, B. (1996). Informed consent: Process and clinical issues. *Oncology Nursing Forum, 23,* 507-514.

Burr, W. R., Hill, R., Nye, F. I., & Reiss, I. R. (Eds.). (1979). *Contemporary theories about the family* (Vols. 1 & 2). New York: Free Press.

Campbell, J. C., & Bunting, S. (1991). Voices and paradigms: Perspectives on critical feminist theory in nursing. *Advances in Nursing Science, 13*(3), 1-15.

Consensus Conference on Guidelines for Adolescent Health Research. (1995). Guidelines for adolescent health research. *Journal of Adolescent Health, 17,* 264-269.

Cromwell, R. E., & Peterson, G. W. (1981). Multisystem-multimethod assessment: A framework. In E. Filsinger & R. A. Lewis (Eds.), *Assessing marriage: New behavioral approaches* (pp. 38-54). Beverly Hills, CA: Sage.

Daly, K. (1992). The fit between qualitative research and characteristics of families. In J. F. Gilgun, K. Daly, & G. Handel (Eds.), *Qualitative methods in family research* (pp. 1-11). Newbury Park, CA: Sage.

Deatrick, J. A., Faux, S. A., & Moore, C. M. (1993). The contribution of qualitative research to the study of families' experiences with childhood illness. In S. L. Feetham, S. B. Meister, J. M. Bell, & C. L. Gilliss (Eds.), *The nursing of families. Theory/research/education/practice* (pp. 61-69). Newbury Park, CA: Sage.

Demi, A. S., & Warren, N. A. (1995). Issues in conducting research with vulnerable families. *Western Journal of Nursing Research, 17,* 188-202.

Feetham, S. L. (1991). Conceptual and methodological issues in research of families. In A. L. Whall & J. Fawcett (Eds.), *Family theory development in nursing: State of the science and art* (pp. 55-68). Philadelphia: F. A. Davis.

Gates, M. F. (1994). Caring behaviors experienced by couples during a hysterectomy. In M. Leininger (Ed.), *Discovery and uses in clinical and community nursing* (pp. 71-85). Detroit, MI: Wayne State University Press.

Gates, M. F., & Lackey, N. R. (1998). Youngster caring for adults with cancer. *Image: Journal of Nursing Scholarship, 30,* 11-15.

Gates, M. F., Lackey, N. R., & White, M. R. (1995). Needs of hospice and clinic patients with cancer. *Cancer Practice, 3,* 226-232.

Gilgun, J. F. (1992). Definitions, methodologies, and methods in qualitative family research. In J. F. Gilgun, K. Daly, & G. Handel (Eds.), *Qualitative methods in family research.* (pp. 22-40). Newbury Park, CA: Sage.

Gilgun, J. F., Daly, K., & Handel, G. (1992). *Qualitative methods in family research.* Newbury Park, CA: Sage.

Gubrium, J. F., & Holstein, J. A. (1991). *What is a family?* Mountain View, CA: Mayfield.

Gubrium, J. F., & Holstein, J. A. (1993). Phenomenology, ethnomethodology, and family discourse. In P. G. Boss, W. J. Doherty, R. LaRossa, W. R. Schumm, & S. K. Steinmetz (Eds.), *Sourcebook of family theories and methods: A contextual approach* (pp. 651-672). New York: Plenum.

Handel, G. (1992). The qualitative tradition in family research. In J. F. Gilgun, K. Daly, & G. Handel (Eds.), *Qualitative methods in family research* (pp. 12-21). Newbury Park, CA: Sage.

Harrington, V., Lackey, N. R. & Gates, M. F. (1996). Needs of caregivers of clinic and hospice cancer patients, *Cancer Nursing, 19,* 118-125.

Johnson, M. A. (1998). Who is the family? In B. Vaughan-Cole, M. A. Johnson, J. A. Malone, & B. L. Walker (Eds.), *Family nursing practice* (pp. 3-18). Philadelphia: W.B. Saunders.

Lackey, N. R., & Gates, M. F. (1994). *Family needs study: Final report.* Memphis, TN: Sigma Theta Tau, Beta Theta Chapter-at-Large.

LaRossa, R., Bennett, L. A., & Gelles, R. J. (1981). Ethical dilemmas in qualitative family research. *Journal of Marriage and the Family, 43,* 303-313.

LaRossa, R., & Wolf, J. H. (1985). On qualitative family research. *Journal of Marriage and the Family, 47,* 531-541.

Malone, J. A. (1997). Family adaptation: Adult sons with long-term physical or mental illnesses. *Issues in Mental Health Nursing, 18,* 351-363.

Moriarty, H. J., & Cotroneo, M. (1993). Sampling issues and family research: Recruitment and sampling strategies. In S. L. Feetham, S. B. Meister, J. M. Bell, & C. L. Gilliss (Eds.), *The nursing of families: Theory/research/education/practice* (pp. 79-89). Newbury Park, CA: Sage.

Murphy, S. O. (1992). Using multiple forms of family data: Identifying pattern and meaning in sibling-infant relationships. In J. F. Gilgun, K. Daly, & G. Handel (Eds.), *Qualitative methods in family research* (pp. 146-171). Newbury Park, CA: Sage.

Rosenblatt, P. C., & Fischer, L. R. (1993). Qualitative family research. In P. G. Boss, W. J. Doherty, R. LaRossa, W. R. Schumm, & S. K. Steinmetz (Eds.), *Sourcebook of family theories and methods: A contextual approach* (pp. 167-177). New York: Plenum.

Thomas, R. (1987). Methodological issues and problems in family health care research. *Journal of Marriage and the Family, 49,* 65-70.

Uphold, C. R., & Strickland, O. L. (1989). Issues related to the unit of analysis of family nursing research. *Western Journal of Nursing Research, 11,* 405-417.

Walsh, D. J. (1998). Generating data. In M. E. Grave & D. J. Walsh (Eds.), *Studying children in context: Theories, methods, and ethics* (pp. 91-128). Thousand Oaks, CA: Sage.

Whall, A. L., & Fawcett, J. (1991). The family as a focal phenomenon in nursing. In A. L. Whall & J. Fawcett (Eds.), *Family theory development in nursing: State of the science and art* (pp. 7-29). Philadelphia: F. A. Davis.

Yarrow, L. J. (1960). Interviewing children. In P. H. Mussen (Ed.), *Handbook of research in child development* (pp. 561-602). New York: Wiley.

5

Qualitative Research Experience With a Community Focus

Joyce V. Zerwekh
with Lee SmithBattle, Margaret Diekemper,
and Mary Ann Drake

This chapter briefly describes many of the disciplines conducting qualitative community studies and the kind of qualitative community studies conducted by nursing. The ethical and methodological issues around observing and studying vulnerable populations are briefly addressed. I lament that few authors have shared their subjective experiences of doing such qualitative work. The heart of the chapter illustrates experiences of conducting community-based qualitative investigations. Emphasizing my own work and that of SmithBattle, Drake, and Diekemper (1997, 1999a, 1999b), two extended descriptions of studying the expertise of nurses who work with vulnerable families and groups in the community are presented. The chapter concludes with comparing and contrasting these two different paths to the study of community health nurse expertise.

QUALITATIVE COMMUNITY INVESTIGATORS

Qualitative community research is being pursued by an ever-expanding number of scholars, including those in the behavioral sciences of anthropology, social psychology, political science, gerontology, and sociology and those in practice disciplines, including education from preschool to university and technical studies, social work, physical therapy, occupational therapy, community medicine and public health, rehabilitation medicine, health education, marketing, women's studies, community organizing, organizational development, addiction studies, criminal justice, and applied ethics. Qualitative inquiry seeks to understand the experience of people living, working, and going to school in their natural living environments, as well as to understand the experience of the professionals working with those people. A community may be defined as a group of individuals composing a social or political unit or a group living or interacting (or both) within particular geographical boundaries. Many times, qualitative community research focuses on activities in the community environment outside of institutions. Sometimes, the focus is understanding the entire community as an entity; focus groups are appropriately used for qualitative community assessment (Stevens, 1996).

Qualitative community health nursing research selects subgroups of informants as representative of vulnerable families, communities, or populations. Often, the research seeks to understand the world and lived experience of people whose socioeconomic status, immigration status, racial and ethnic background, social behavior, stigmatized health conditions, or chronic disability place them on the margins of society, outside the mainstream. For instance, qualitative studies have sought to understand the experiences of the homeless (Francis, 1992; Hatton, 1997), those living with AIDS and those facing multiple losses due to AIDS-related deaths (Carmack, 1992; Dolan & Nokes, 1992), youth struggling with issues around drug dependence (Anderson, 1996), diverse immigrant groups (D'Avanzo, Frye, & Froman, 1994; MacKinnon, Gien, & Durst, 1996), those heavily burdened by family caregiving (Boland & Sims, 1996; Grant & Davis, 1997; Stetz & Brown, 1997), and the vulnerable elderly (Krothe, 1997; Porter, 1994). Community health nursing qualitative investigators seek to understand the health-related experiences of diverse ethnic groups, including African American women (Banks-Wallace, 1988; Bolla, DeJoseph, Norbeck, & Smith, 1996) and Native Americans at risk for diabetes (Jacobson et al., 1998) Likewise, as shown in the following discussion, community health nursing scholars seek to understand the world and experience of nurses working with these vulnerable groups.

UNTOLD EXPERIENCE

The human experience of doing qualitative research tends to be snuffed out in the writing of papers for publication. The untold stories of investigator experience include the ethical and intellectual and emotional challenges and joys in collecting, interpreting, and writing up the research.

Demi and Warren (1995) review the literature on ethical issues in studying at-risk populations. The literature examines issues of informed consent, risk for informants versus any perceived benefits, and confidentiality. They consider the following ethical questions: What is the responsibility to break confidentiality if the investigator witnesses child or elder abuse and neglect? Is observed parenting behavior abusive or culturally appropriate? Is it right for the investigator to bring up problems in the interview without any expectation of their being fixed? What about informant and investigator stress when sensitive or embarrassing material is disclosed? When investigators are from mainstream culture, avoiding racist, sexist, and classist perspectives are major issues. In addition, researchers may have realistic concerns for their personal safety in crime-ridden neighborhoods.

Methodological issues in conducting studies with vulnerable families in community include recruitment and retention of participants and appropriateness of the interview questions for people living outside the mainstream (Demi & Warren, 1995). For instance, stress among 120 refugee Cambodian women was explored in one study by involving a trusted community leader to provide entry to households and to translate. The subjects were potentially resistant and therefore accessed by network sampling. They were told that the study was not related to the government and that they were free to refuse consent (D'Avanzo et al., 1994). There may be significant barriers to truthfulness when other household members are overhearing interviews or when the interview may reveal illegal or socially stigmatized activities. For instance, homeless women protested audio taping of their responses to questions about their health because they considered their problems to be shameful (Hatton, 1997).

In contrast, Hutchinson, Wilson, and Wilson (1994) noted that vulnerable community informants can experience great benefit from sensitive interviewing by engaged listeners. Storytelling can heal and give participants a feeling of being validated. Exploration of difficult experiences can help them gain a new perspective and feel empowered. "In-depth research interviews can give a voice to the voiceless" (p. 164).

What about the joys and struggles of interpretation and writing? Harry Wolcott (1994) describes a major challenge of qualitative research as "transforming unruly experience into an 'authoritative written account' " (p. 10). I could find no community-focused research article that dared acknowledge the affective experience of turning chaos into order. Munhall (1994) proclaims laughing a little and crying a little at researcher experiences in phenomenology. She acknowledges that exploring the affective emotive domain requires that "you must evaluate your capacity for self-revelation and the display of emotion" (p. 70). I particularly liked the openness to surprise that she describes as a critical dimension of phenomenology: "Literally leave your beliefs at home and find out how others structure their reality; how others perceive their world; be truly unknowing so that you can be open to variations and even contradictions of your cherished beliefs" (p. 84). Dare we make ourselves this vulnerable and undertake to have a "beginner's mind" to understand the human experience of others? If not, we continue to "discover" our preconceptions!

The following sections detail two investigative experiences, undertaken in Washington State and Missouri, to discover and name the expert practice of community health nurses. Other relevant studies are briefly overviewed, and the chapter concludes by comparing and contrasting the two investigations.

DISCOVERING THE EXPERTISE OF COMMUNITY HEALTH NURSES

Intending to depict my own and colleagues' human experience of doing research, the lens is now narrowed to the qualitative study of nurses caring in community. Hopefully, discussion of this single focus will provoke the reader to consider implications for the entire area of qualitative community research.

To my knowledge, I was the first to describe expert community health nursing practice in detail, based on qualitative study, and to develop a practice model. The next section explores my research experience.

Does Expert Nursing Practice Actually Exist?

A 9-year, intense immersion in the practice of home health and hospice nursing was the foundation for my studying first public health nursing and later hospice nursing expertise. I worked as a home health nurse and coordinator from 1977 to 1979. In 1979, my colleagues and I launched Seattle's first home visiting hospice program at Hospice of Seattle, and I later coordinated the development of Seattle's first inpatient hospice unit. I had been working with exceptional nurse colleagues, and we accomplished the exceptional for suffering people. Then in 1986, I walked into the university to teach hospice and community health nursing. In the university setting, I was shocked to encounter great skepticism about practicing nurses. Indeed, whenever nursing practice or documentation was observed by academics, they were consistently found inadequate. To me as a newcomer, the underlying assumption appeared to be that practicing nurses were ineffective as a whole group!

Convinced that expert practice knowledge did exist and that I had seen it and heard it and felt it from nurse colleagues, it was a great joy to discover Patricia Benner's (1984) description of excellence and power in clinical nursing practice, *From Novice to Expert*. Based on qualitative interpretation of expert hospital nurse interviews, she named previously unacclaimed nursing competencies and used anecdotes to illustrate and explain them. I could not have agreed more fully with her writing,

> Our language needs to be enriched by a new immersion in the actual practice of nursing. The linear ideal that theory must be generated first and then applied to nursing has given us a deficit view of nursing practice, allowing us only to see the gaps. (p. 219)

That indeed was what I was finding in academia—a deficit view that highlighted gaps.

This failure to recognize clinical wisdom is as old as Western civilization. The virtues of theoretical wisdom have persistently been elevated over practical wisdom. Even though they are professors in a practice discipline, until recently, university nursing faculty have downplayed practice wisdom.

Meanwhile, in the late 1980s, Patricia Benner was not the only one saying there was much to learn from clinician stories. In *The Call of Stories,* Robert Coles (1989) proposed that stories of particular clinical experiences have much to teach us. Reviewing public health nursing knowledge development, Hamilton and Bush (1988) proposed that practice could be elucidated by examining stories of historical and contemporary public health nurses. But I'm getting ahead of my own story. Somewhere in the process of exploring Benner's (1984) research and qualitative research methodology, I made a decision to focus outside hospice nursing for my initial study. I was deeply embedded in hospice practice, teaching, writing, and speaking. I felt my opinions and prejudgments were too strong. I felt I "knew" what hospice nursing competency was and that I needed to turn my attention elsewhere where I could have a beginner's mind.

Making Public Health Nursing Visible

Public health nursing in the home was an appealing alternative. Public health "field nurses" work with high-risk mothers and children and are employed by local government-funded public health departments. Investigating public health nursing would expand my knowledge of so-called womb-to-tomb nursing in the community. I came to the field as a novice, with the exception of my own student experience visiting alone an African American family with a new baby. My ignorance in that situation had been overwhelming. They had multiple children; I knew almost nothing about children. They referred to each other as "brothers" and "sisters" and "mothers," and I never figured out who was whom. But they were gracious enough not to turn me away at the door. Twenty-five years later, I literally had no opinions or prejudgments about public health nursing practice other than that I suspected it was worthwhile and very challenging.

Review of the public health nursing literature soon revealed that home visiting was actually a nearly invisible practice that occurred behind closed doors, was poorly articulated in literature, and was poorly funded. Surprisingly akin to hospice home nursing of the dying, public health nurse home visits to childbearing families relied on exquisite communication skills, with teaching as its central purpose. The need to more clearly document this practice was proclaimed by Erickson (1987) as local health department nursing positions and programs were being cut because of the "inability to articulate the pivotal role of public health nursing in the delivery of essential health services" (p. 204). Well, this looked like it could be a relevant study! Public health nurses needed to document their expertise and the critical services they rendered to ensure their continued their existence!

The question of what method to use was a major challenge. From what I could see in the limited qualitative research texts available at that time, I could "do" ethnography, phenomenology, or grounded theory. I was continually drawn to the qualitative approach designed by Benner. In 1983 and 1984, she elucidated her unique synthesis of phenomenology and selected application of the constant comparative method of Glaser and Strauss's (1967) grounded theory. She stated that she was using hermeneutics to interpret the transcribed text of nurses' story. To discover content and meanings, she identified exemplars, interpreted them for recurring themes, and then validated her interpretation by practice experts.

I decided to describe my research method as *eclectic phenomenological,* inspired throughout by Patricia Benner (1984) blazing a trail before me. From the first nursing textbook on grounded theory (Chenitz & Swanson, 1986) and early texts reviewing qualitative methods (Leininger, 1985; Munhall & Oiler Boyd, 1986), it was clear to me that I was not ready to embark on substantive theory development that is the end goal of grounded theory. However, the stepwise data analysis methods of grounded theory were the best articulated in the literature at the time. Although phenomenological methods were hard to get a handle on in the late 1980s, my aim was clearly phenomenological: to describe the practice experience and meaning of that experience as lived by public health nurses practicing with maternal and child clients in the home. To uncover subjective realities of practicing nurses, I would scrutinize the narrative text of their stories.

To explore postpositivist qualitative inquiry, I studied Lincoln and Guba (1985). Consistent with this view of reality, the investigator and the investigated mutually shape one another, and the inquirer's frame of reference always affects the inquiry. One of the greatest strengths that I brought to the inquiry was my ability to listen attentively without interruption. This lesson I learned through 7 years of listening to dying people and their families. Failure to listen without interrupting and leading informants are serious pitfalls of qualitative research. In contrast, I knew how to be still. I also brought to the investigation 22 years of nursing practice and education, including significant publishing experience. I had spent much of my career trying to discern underlying patterns of experience to explain them to students or in conceptual writing for journals and texts. My interpretation in particular was informed by rather a strong foundation in reading nursing ethics and biomedical ethics literature. It was through these frames of reference that I viewed the transcribed text.

Two interview questions guided my questions to informants: "Tell about one or more anecdotes when you believe that your home visiting really made a difference in the outcome of a family at risk." And "Describe your clinical examples that represent the essence of your work in public health nursing." I interviewed an arbitrarily predetermined sample of 30 expert public health nurses who had 5 or more years of experience and whose supervisors identified as experts to whom other public health nurses turned for clinical advice. The 30 nurses had a mean age of 45 years old with a mean of 20 years in nursing and 14 in public health. They came from five health departments in western Washington state; all but one held a bachelor's degree in nursing. They were rural, urban, and suburban nurses largely visiting impoverished families.

The interview process itself was revealing. First of all, the nurses had difficulty telling stories with detail and color. Used to presenting brief case reports, they tended to reduce the story to a skeleton, which then had to be fleshed out by asking for what happened next and how did they feel and what were they thinking and what did they do and what did they think it all meant. One nurse was unable to speak in story format. Urged beyond reductionism, many of the 29 others came to speak poetically and in metaphor through 95 stories. For instance, to locate families, they "sniff them out and track them down." They "get a line on them" and "put out feelers." To detect what's going on, they describe themselves as detectives looking for clues and gardeners weeding out what is really happening. They "smell violence." In timing interventions, they refer to "windows in time" and use gardening metaphors about soil too hard to plant seeds, seeds washing away, ready soil, and sprouting seed.

Despite this eloquence, I was often saddened by the nurse's self-deprecation, a humility that I have since come to term "suicidal." They would put their work down by saying, "I just hung in there with them," or "It was just common sense," or "I really didn't do anything." If we nurses cannot acknowledge the strength of our own practice, how can we expect outsiders—citizens, policymakers, other health professionals—to do so? I have since described this downplaying of practice knowledge as "practice ignorance" and defined it as the inability to articulate the knowledge needed to practice.

After they had told their stories, the nurses consistently shared their pleasure at having been heard. They could recognize their own expertise as their stories unfolded. As my experience with interviews grew and the power of the stories became evident, I puzzled over the requirements of protecting their privacy as human subjects. As is standard practice to maintain confidentiality, number codes were substituted for each nurse's name, which was, from that moment on, known only to myself. The consent process ensured these nurses confidentiality and anonymity, but at times, I have regretted that they therefore cannot be named and celebrated for their wisdom.

I took handwritten notes while taping each nurse's interview so that I began to compare my notes for repeating themes very early in the process. My scrutiny of the narratives focused on persistently asking the question, "What is the nurse really doing here?" Tapes were sent for transcription in clumps, and when the first group returned, I had the challenge of learning Ethnograph software. Throughout my naming and renaming of competencies and their dimensions, I sought to use the nurses' own words and idioms (emic perspective) rather than imposing more academic-sounding categories. For instance, they repeatedly spoke about themselves as detectives searching for evidence, and so I described holistic assessment as the "detecting" competency. I ended up with two domains of nursing competency, Family Caregiving and Nurse Preserving.

Within Family Caregiving, I had a list of 15 nursing competencies and labored to arrange them in linear outline format, with subcompetencies listed underneath. Here is where I unconsciously left the domain of interpretive phenomenology in seeking to understand the relationships between each competency category. I could not figure out how to order the list of competencies; everything overlapped. Trying to discern order and connections, I drew many versions of a so-called *mind map* on my kitchen table. I had an opportunity to seek counsel with Dr. Mel Haberman, nurse researcher at the Fred Hutchinson Cancer Research Center in Seattle, and showed him my crude diagrams drawn in search of order. Mel suggested that what I had drawn was a nursing model. So I discovered what I had not set out to find. A few days later, the "Public Health Nursing Family Caregiving Model" was born, to be followed several years later by her sister, the "Hospice Family Caregiving Model" (Zerwekh, 1995).

In the center of the circular Family Caregiving Model, I drew "Encouraging Family Self-Help" and called it the hub around which other contributing competencies came together. I have since realized that grounded theorists would call this a Basic Social Process, the underlying social process for which they search as the basis of the phenomenon being studied. I accidently discovered a Basic Social Process when I wasn't looking for one. It simply appeared in the center of my model because encouraging self-help was the underlying theme of *every* expert public health nurse's story.

The credibility of my family caregiving model and competencies was strengthened by three checks with members of stakeholding groups, recommended by Lincoln and Guba (1985). The preliminary model and competencies were revised and reshaped through dialogue with a separate group of practicing public health nurses and with a group of faculty peers. In a final check with informants, all 30 nurse experts were sent a written summary and interpretation. Their suggestions and ideas were integrated into the final model. In my hospice study, I would invite feedback earlier in model development.

Like many researchers, I had a problem with uncovering data that didn't fit with my initial purpose, which was to describe public health nursing competencies. Whole sections of interviews were irrelevant to this purpose because they focused on difficulties and failures going alone into homes where hardship and adversity prevailed. In my search for victory stories, I set them aside. But how long can you turn your head away and pretend you just do not see? Reexamining these discarded stories of hardship at the very end of my research process, I decided that they were about Expert Public Health Nurse Preserving and named three recurring themes: struggling with adversity, confronting violence, and preserving nurse well-being. Ironically, the first article to be published about my research was a summary of my initially unwanted results. Lucie Kelly, then editor of *Nursing Outlook,* was immediately engaged by the color and power of the stories. I was honored by her excitement and support. She even changed the title from my proposed dry academic one to the compelling headline, "At the Expense of Their Souls" (Zerwekh, 1991a). It was derived from the words of one of my informants:

> This past year I really haven't been able to make a difference. It's at the expense of my soul. . . . I'm not willing to live only in the world of high risk, CPS, sex abuse, drug addiction. There's not enough time to get replenished. (p. 60)

I was surprised when colleagues told me that this article was banned in several health departments when first published. Consultants and educators brought copies in for staff nurses to read and discuss, and supervisors declined to distribute the material because it was "too disturbing and not a problem in our town." So I had not wanted to look at this reality initially, and neither did it settle well with some nursing managers.

Following this initial article, I was able to publish my model and descriptions of practice expertise in several refereed and nonrefereed journals (Zerwekh, 1991b, 1992a, 1992b). I have been privileged to present my work and dialogue with public health nurses all over the United States and Canada. My public health nursing study became a foundation for my own next task: articulating the practice wisdom of home-visiting hospice nurses.

MAKING HOSPICE NURSING VISIBLE

About 2 years after completing the public health nursing study, I decided I was ready to complete a similar study of hospice nursing. I returned for a summer and fall to the practice and wrote stories of my most memorable visits. Several of these narratives I later included with the stories of other hospice nurses. My data was drawn from multiple sources, broader than the prior study because of my own wide reading in the field and years of practice experience.

Experts were defined in the same way, and questions simply substituted hospice nursing for public health nursing. I collected stories from 31 hospice nursing experts and included my own stories. Responding nurses demonstrated similar levels of humility and tendencies to put themselves down, with statements such as, "I really don't do that much. The families do all the work."

I sought to examine the transcribed narratives by discarding preconceived categories. Each interview was documented first in handwritten notes, which were coded with tentative names soon after the meeting. Preliminary code names expanded over time to a maximum of 27 nursing competency categories. In the midst of my investigation, after interviewing 18 nurses and before I became too committed to conclusions, I convened 10 of my hospice nurse experts for 2 hours. They critiqued preliminary competency names and a preliminary computer drawing seeking to visualize how the competencies were all connected with "being there" at the center. The group struggled with how to depict multiple overlapping relationships visually. The diagram progressed from geometric circles, which were strongly rejected, to a daisy, and finally to a deeply rooted tree. After their input and examination and reexamination of all 32 nurses' stories, the competency categories were condensed to 10.

Soon after the focus group meeting, the Hospice Nursing Family Caregiving Model was generated in final form. "Sustaining Oneself" roots the tree in position and makes it possible for the nurse to care. The trunk connects the roots to the branches and represents the interpersonal "Connecting" competency. Connecting is the process of joining in relationship with family and patient. "Encouraging Choice" extends the trunk upward out of "Connecting," and all other competencies extend as limbs from that center. Final refinement of competency descriptions was provided by written feedback from 14 of the nurse informants.

I particularly enjoyed publishing the organic model and some of the ideas from this research (Zerwekh, 1995). I loved portraying the integral nature of caring for self, so essential that the whole tree would fall if the nurse does not give attention to herself. Many of the nurses' "Connecting" stories were striking examples of the poorly understood therapeutic dance. The expert, rigorous efforts to practice "Comforting" were vividly illustrated: "I feel like I'm making a little custom-made suit every time I go on a visit. Tailor the plan to where they're at with physical and psychological comfort."

SUBSEQUENT STUDIES TO
ARTICULATE PRACTICE WISDOM

My public health study and the hospice nursing studies have provided practice models and shared conceptual language for practicing nurses to develop a clear mental picture of their practice wisdom and to be better able to make their practice visible to fellow professionals, students, managers, policy makers, and the public. However, Barbara Robertson Green (1993), who interviewed eight practicing New Zealand public health nurses, has uncovered a contradiction at the very heart of the challenge to document invisible and taken-for-granted practice:

> The paradox between the necessity of working hard to increase visibility . . . contrasts with the secrecy and confidentiality required for much of their work. Public health nurses note that aspects of their work are unpalatable and difficult for society to contemplate. (p. 109)

We are seeking to make visible what society would rather not see or know!

Appleton (1996), Byrd (1997), Chalmers (1992), Leipert (1996), Paavilainen and Astedt-Kurki (1997), and Reutter and Ford (1996) have completed noteworthy qualitative studies of nursing practice in the community that were published after mine. Little is preserved in their published papers to help us understand the human experience of these investigators as they were challenged to transform their unruly data. The requirements of academic writing continue to require linear, objective, technical accounts. Although this research is grounded in the power of story and dramatic practice experience, the feelings and flesh have been excised for publication. The poetry and challenge of inquiry is deliberately put aside in the telling.

Applying interpretive phenomenology, SmithBattle and colleagues (Smith-Battle, Diekemper, & Drake, 1997; SmithBattle, Drake, et al., 1997) have engaged in collaborative study of community health nursing, which I believe constitutes the next wave of qualitative work to elucidate community health nursing practice wisdom. With 25 community health nurse informants, they have conducted individual and small group interviews, and they have completed field observations, including home visits, clinic activities, case management, and community meetings. I have asked them to compare and contrast their research experience with mine.

* * * * *

From the Three Professors from St. Louis: SmithBattle, Diekemper, and Drake:

That Joyce Zerwekh has brought such high-profile visibility to public health nursing practice attests to her engagement with the data and her skills as interviewer and writer. Equally noteworthy is her openness and willingness to engage others—us, in this instance—in a dialogue about the qualitative research experience and how our particular findings differ in some important ways from hers. We should acknowledge at the outset that our approach to uncovering public health nursing expertise differed in two ways from Zerwekh's. First, we were not as new to the practice as Zerwekh describes herself. Rather, as colleagues, our experience encompassed a combined 63 years of public health nursing, which provided an important foundation for the research. Our collective experience included both family and population-focused practice with diverse populations, including migrant farm workers, immigrant-refugee groups, teenage mothers, high-risk families, and the elderly.

Second, because Lee SmithBattle had been mentored in interpretive phenomenology by Patricia Benner and others at the University of California at San Francisco and Berkeley, we did not have to learn research methodology on our own and from the ground up. In fact, we studied the philosophical background of interpretive phenomenology before beginning the study to have the best possible grasp of the notions of practice and practical knowledge. This experiential and philosophical background prepared us, as we will later discuss, to maintain fidelity to the data and to nursing practice. From our perspective, Zerwekh entered the research arena under what we personally consider to be adverse research conditions. In spite of these circumstances, Zerwekh has sensitively detailed the uncelebrated work of public health nurses (PHNs), and her widely celebrated publications have been largely validated and applauded in the PHN community.

Camaraderie and Celebration

The seeds for our enthusiasm for public health nursing and nursing stories were first planted when we met as PHNs at a neighborhood health center. Our nursing practice with vulnerable populations was supported and modeled by Edna Dell Weinel, the executive director of the agency and an expert PHN. A marvelous storyteller herself, she has mentored each of us throughout our careers by example, story, advice, and consultation. It was without reservation that we asked her to be involved with the study, knowing that her 40-plus years of PHN experience would be invaluable in analyzing nurses' stories. We could now proudly boast of over a century of public health nursing experience! She welcomed the opportunity to study both expert and beginner practice with the hope that the findings would help nurses shape their future practice. So it was with camaraderie and enthusiasm that we embarked on the study.

As we began, we followed Benner's example (1984; Benner, Tanner, & Chesla, 1996) by first conducting small group interviews in pairs with nurses of similar experiential levels to hone our interviewing skills and to encourage clinical storytelling among peers (See Benner, 1994b, pp. 109-110, for discussion of the role of group interviews in eliciting clinical narratives). After the group interviews were completed, we met with nurses individually to interview them and observe them in their routine activities in homes, clinics, on the phone, or in the community. The field observations and debriefing of nurses provided an avenue to situate us in each nurse's practice and helped us to notice and explore particularly pervasive, taken-for-granted aspects of expertise. Seeing everyday aspects of practice first-hand often led us to pose new questions on the spot after debriefing sessions with the nurse and during future interviews or data analysis. This process ultimately helped us to uncover unnoticed aspects of practice.

Soon after initiating data collection, we began monthly meetings with our mentor to analyze nurses' stories. Data analysis proved to be an invigorating dialogue moving back and forth from one clinical story to another, allowing each story to deepen our understanding, challenge our preconceptions, and flesh out some of the nuances of practice. For example, it was only in reading nurses' stories of "breaking the rules" that we came to appreciate this hidden and effective aspect of practice in which nurses go beyond bureaucratic rules and agency policies to address the needs of families or communities (Drake, SmithBattle, & Diekemper, 1998). In analyzing stories of population-focused practice, we uncovered distinctions between "natural" and "intentional" practice and began, and only began, to detect the key role of support and supervision in shaping a nurse's participation and skill in community practice (Diekemper, SmithBattle, & Drake, 1999a, 1999b). We also began to notice in story after story how the expert's responsiveness of self enabled her to gain a situated understanding of clients' lives and to cultivate clients' strengths and connections to a responsive community (SmithBattle, Drake, & Diekemper, 1997).

Articulation Versus Model Building

From the outset, we had no intention of discovering a theory or developing a model to represent practice. As Benner et al. (1992) have made clear, the clinical world is a practical, not a theoretical, world that necessarily eludes formalization and scientific model building. Given our phenomenological perspective, our purpose was to articulate practice; that is, to make the skillful know-how of PHNs, as well as the constraints and supports to excellent practice, more accessible and visible (Benner, 1994a). As Zerwekh herself noted earlier, whole aspects of public health nursing practice did not fit with her purpose or emerging model. To her credit, ignoring discrepant data was recognized as problematic and moved her to reexamine and make sense of the data—although in ways that departed significantly from our interpretation of similar data. Like the participants profiled in Zerwekh's (1991a) article, nurses in our study also described coming face to face with great suffering, extreme vulnerability, and chaotic situations. But it was their varied responses to these situations, based on experience and supervision, that helped us to further illuminate the expert's responsiveness. For example, early in our analysis, we were struck by experts' language of hope and possibility in situations that would cause many to despair. Their sense of hope had been cultivated by long-term relationships and a "big picture" perspective gained by knowing families and communities over significant periods of time. The complex interweaving of clients' life experiences helped nurses to recognize how human lives are always situated, rather than chosen, and ultimately shaped nurses' judgment of outcomes and possible actions. The experts' language and engagement in the situation differed radically from the few demoralized nurses we identified as being disengaged from their practice (See Rubin, 1996). It was these nurses who reacted to clients' situations as futile and who distanced themselves, sometimes blaming the clients for their own circumstances. Beginners, on the other hand, encountered what for them were overwhelming situations and sometimes rushed in to rescue the family. However, their own accounts described how good supervision encouraged them to become engaged with so-called difficult families in ways that were productive for the family.

Like Zerwekh, we found that nurses sometimes initially spoke in generalities about their practice until it was clear that we were interested, not in generalities, but in the most obvious details of practice that are only revealed in narratives. We were not dismayed to find that nurses needed coaching to tell stories or that they would make seemingly self-deprecating comments, such as "I just did it." We expected experts to speak a language of humility and common sense, because clinical expertise becomes second nature, and the most taken-for-granted aspects of practice escape attention and elude theories and scientific models. Experts' common sense language reflects the nature of expertise itself, such that experts "just" do what they do without fanfare or publicity. Nurses also perhaps dismiss the value of clinical storytelling because academics and administrators have rarely promoted clinical narratives as a legitimate source of knowledge development. But as Zerwekh and our team discovered, public storytelling powerfully validates practice. A nurse with 20 years of experience made this clear when she said,

> Sometimes, when I hear myself talk about these stories, it makes me very proud to be a nurse all over again. Because sometimes in your everyday work with the large caseload you have, you get so busy just trying to get through your everyday work, you forget about all the good things that you've done because you're just getting it done.

The Future

Although we are by no means complacent about the cultural forces that devalue public health and nursing practice in general, the finding from the two studies just described have expanded our learning and teaching of students and have reminded us of the commitment and passion that expert PHNs bring to the field. We have also been encouraged to find nurses across the spectrum of experience who directly grasp the relevance of the stories for their own practice. Although the confidentiality of nurse participants was assumed and the numbers were small, we felt an obligation to return to agencies to share the study findings with the participants (who remained unnamed) and their peers. During these sessions, nurses engaged in an active dialogue, uncovering additional aspects of practice as they participated in public storytelling. We were also heartened to find health departments and innovative practice sites that were committed to strengthening the PHN tradition after a period of retrenchment (SmithBattle, Diekemper, & Drake, 1997). We are about to begin a second, longitudinal study to better understand the constraints and supports to the development of expertise. We expect that such qualitative findings will be available for immediate translation into practice, validating the relevance of the research and confirming that clinical practice is a neglected but rich repository of knowledge.

* * * * *

CONTRAST AND UNITY

The St. Louis team and I (Zerwekh) both enthusiastically confirm the rich practice knowledge of community health nurses. However, they traveled some different paths and made some strikingly different assumptions. SmithBattle and colleagues completed their work approximately 5 years later than I, when community qualitative inquiry had matured. My work established groundwork for theirs. While they were a team of investigators in constant collaboration, I was a single investigator. SmithBattle and colleagues had direct experience as PHNs with mostly young, vulnerable families, whereas my community practice experience was with the elderly and dying. SmithBattle and colleagues had studied phenomenology in depth and were mentored by a nationally known phenomenological nursing researcher. SmithBattle used both participant observation and interview; I used interview alone. Both affirmed the meaning of storytelling experience for their informants. I was more troubled by nurses' humility and inability to explain their practice. Both discovered many previously undiscussed dimensions of community health nursing that continue to contribute to the body of practice knowledge. SmithBattle and colleagues adhere to a philosophical framework that eschews theoretical models, whereas I developed a model as a way to visualize and explain practice dimensions. That model has been replicated and developed through other scholars' work, particularly in many graduate studies, and used in agencies to develop standards of practice. Many paths applying diverse methods and perspectives lead to the development of comprehensive practice knowledge. I hope more investigators will join us on the road.

REFERENCES

Anderson, N. L. R. (1996). Decisions about substance abuse among adolescents in juvenile detention. *Image: The Journal of Nursing Scholarship, 28,* 65-70.

Appleton, J. V. (1996). Working with vulnerable families: A health visiting perspective. *Journal of Advanced Nursing, 23,* 912-918.

Banks-Wallace, J. (1998). Emancipatory potential of storytelling in a group. *Image: Journal of Nursing Scholarship, 30,* 17-22.

Benner, P. (1983). Uncovering the knowledge embedded in clinical practice. *Image: Journal of Nursing Scholarship, 15,* 36-41.

Benner, P. (1984). *From novice to expert: Excellence and power in clinical nursing practice.* Redwood City, CA: Addison-Wesley.

Benner, P. (1994a). The role of articulation in understanding practice and excellence as sources of knowledge in clinical nursing. In J. Tully & D. M. Weinstock (Eds), *Philosophy in a time of pluralism: Perspectives on the philosophy of Charles Taylor* (pp. 136-155). New York: Cambridge University Press.

Benner, P. (1994b). The tradition and skill of interpretive phenomenology in studying health, illness, and caring practices. In P. Benner (Ed.), *Interpretive phenomenology: Embodiment, caring, and ethics in health and illness* (pp. 99-127). Thousand Oaks, CA: Sage.

Benner, P. A., Tanner, C. A., & Chesla, C. A. (1992). From beginner to expert: Gaining a differentiated clinical world in critical care nursing. *Advances in Nursing Science, 14,* 13-28.

Benner, P. A., Tanner, C. A., & Chesla, C. A. (1996). *Expertise in nursing practice: Caring, clinical judgment, and ethics.* New York: Springer.

Boland, D. L., & Sims, S. L. (1996). Family caregiving at home as a solitary journey. *Image: Journal of Nursing Scholarship, 28,* 55-58.

Bolla, C. D., DeJoseph, J., Norbeck, J., & Smith, R. (1996). Social support as road map and vehicle: An analysis of data from focus group interviews with a group of African-American women. *Public Health Nursing, 13,* 331-336.

Byrd, M. E. (1997). Child-focused single home visiting. *Public Health Nursing, 14,* 313-322.

Carmack, B. J. (1992). Balancing engagement/detachment in AIDS-related multiple losses. *Image: Journal of Nursing Scholarship, 24,* 9-14.

Chalmers, K. I. (1992). Giving and receiving: An empirically derived theory on health visiting practice. *Journal of Advanced Nursing, 17,* 1317-1325.

Chenitz, W. C., & Swanson, J. M. (1986). *From practice to grounded theory: Qualitative research in nursing.* Menlo Park, CA: Addison-Wesley.

Coles, R. (1989). *The call of stories: Teaching and the moral imagination.* Boston: Houghton Mifflin.

D'Avanzo, C. E., Frye, B., & Froman, R. (1994). Stress in Cambodian refugee families. *Image: Journal of Nursing Scholarship, 26,* 101-105.

Demi, A. S., & Warren, N. A. (1995). Issues in conducting research with vulnerable families. *Western Journal of Nursing Research, 17,* 188-202.

Diekemper, M., SmithBattle, L., & Drake, M. A. (1999a). Bringing the population into focus: A natural development in community health nursing: Part 1. *Public Health Nursing, 16*(1), 3-10.

Diekemper, M., SmithBattle, L., & Drake, M. A. (1999b). Sharpening the focus on populations: An intentional community health nursing approach: Part 2. *Public Health Nursing, 16*(1), 11-16.

Dolan, M., & Nokes, K. M. (1992). Experiences of New York Puerto Rican family members living with AIDS. *Journal of the Association of Nurses in AIDS Care, 3,* 23-28.

Drake, M. A., SmithBattle, L., Diekemper, M. (1998). *Breaking the rules: A hidden and effective aspect of community health nursing practice.* Manuscript in preparation.

Erickson, G. (1987). Public health nursing initiatives: Guideposts for future practice. *Public Health Nursing, 4,* 202-211.

Francis, M. B. (1992). Eight homeless mother's tales. *Image: Journal of Nursing Scholarship, 24,* 111-114.

Glaser B. G., & Strauss, A. (1967). *The discovery of grounded theory.* Chicago: Aldine.

Grant, J. S. & Davis, L. L. (1997). Living with loss: The stroke family caregiver. *Journal of Family Nursing, 3,* 36-56.

Green, B. R. (1993). *Enabling choice: Public Health Nurses' perceptions of their work with children and families.* Unpublished master's thesis, Massey University, New Zealand.

Hamilton, P. A., & Bush, H. A. (1988). Theory development in community health nursing: Issues and recommendations. *Scholarly Inquiry for Nursing Practice, 2,* 145-165.

Hatton, D. C. (1997). Managing health problems among homeless women with children in a transitional shelter. *Image: Journal of Nursing Scholarship, 29,* 33-37.

Hutchinson, S. A., Wilson, M. E., & Wilson, S. (1994). Benefits of participating in research interviews. *Image: Journal of Nursing Scholarship, 26,* 161-164.

Jacobson, S. F., Booton-Hiser, D., Moore, J. H., Edwards, K. A., Pryor, S., & Campbell, J. M. (1998). Diabetes research in an American Indian community. *Image: Journal of Nursing Scholarship, 30,* 161-165.

Krothe, J. S. (1997). Giving voice to elderly people: Community-based long-term care. *Public Health Nursing, 14,* 217-226.

Leininger, M. (1985). *Qualitative research methods in nursing.* New York: Grune & Stratton.

Leipert, B. D. (1996). The value of community health nursing: a phenomenological study of the perceptions of community health nurses. *Public Health Nursing, 13,* 50-57.

Lincoln, Y. S., & Guba, E. G. (1985). *Naturalistic inquiry.* Beverly Hills, CA: Sage.

MacKinnon, M. E., Gien, L., & Durst, D. (1996). Chinese elders speak out: Implications for caregivers. *Clinical Nursing Research, 5,* 326-342.

Munhall, P. L. (1994). *Revisioning phenomenology: Nursing and health science research.* New York: National League for Nursing Press.

Munhall, P. L., & Oiler Boyd, C. J. (1986). *Nursing research: A qualitative perspective.* Norwalk: Appleton-Century-Crofts.

Paavilainen, E., & Astedt-Kurki, P. (1997). The client-nurse relationship as experienced by public health nurses: Toward better collaboration. *Public Health Nursing, 14,* 137-142.

Porter, E. J. (1994). Older widows' experience of living alone at home. *Image: Journal of Nursing Scholarship, 26,* 19-24.

Reutter, L. I., & Ford, J. S. (1996). Perceptions of public health nursing: Views from the field. *Journal of Advanced Nursing, 24,* 7-15.

Rubin, J. (1996). Impediments to the development of clinical knowledge and ethical judgment in critical care nursing. In P. Benner, C. A. Tanner, & C. A. Chesla (Eds.), *Expertise in nursing practice: Caring, clinical judgment, and ethics* (pp. 170-192). New York: Springer.

SmithBattle, L., Diekemper, M., Drake, M. A. (1997, November). *Everything old is new again: Reclaiming the CHN tradition.* Paper presented at the American Public Health Association Meeting, Indianapolis, IN.

SmithBattle, L., Drake, M. A., & Diekemper, M. (1997). The responsive use of self in community health nursing practice. *Advances in Nursing Science, 20,* 75-89.

Stetz, K. M., & Brown, M. A. (1997). Taking care: Caregiving to persons with cancer and AIDS. *Cancer Nursing, 20,* 12-22.

Stevens, P. E. (1996). Focus groups: Collecting aggregate-level data to understand community health phenomena. *Public Health Nursing, 13,* 170-176.

Wolcott, H. (1994). *Transforming qualitative data: Description, analysis, and interpretation.* Thousand Oaks: Sage.

Zerwekh, J. V. (1991a). At the expense of their souls. *Nursing Outlook, 39,* 58-61.

Zerwekh, J. V. (1991b). A family caregiving model for expert public health home visiting. *Nursing Outlook, 39,* 213-217.

Zerwekh, J. V. (1992a). Laying the groundwork for family self help: Locating families, building trust, and building strength. *Public Health Nursing, 9,* 15-21.

Zerwekh, J. V. (1992b). The practice of empowerment and coercion by expert public health nurses. *Image: Journal of Nursing Scholarship, 24,* 101-105.

Zerwekh, J. V. (1995). A family caregiving model for hospice nursing. *The Hospice Journal, 10,* 27-44.

Six Stories of Researcher Experience in Organizational Studies

Personal and Professional Insights

Kimberly D. Elsbach

What the fieldworker learns is how to appreciate the world in a different key. Early experiences and understandings of the world studied (and their representation in fieldnotes) are not data per se but rather primitive approximations of the writer's later knowledge and perspectives of those studied.
—Van Maanen (1985, p. 118)

The Amway study has changed me. I talk about the one study that has changed the way I look at the world, that would be it. First of all, it kind of made me realize the power of giving people hope at kind of a basic level.
—Michael Pratt, personal interview

This essay is about the ongoing process of being a qualitative organizational researcher. In particular, it is about the process of self-definition and self-identification by qualitative organizational researchers (Schlenker, 1986; i.e., how their distinctive and defining attributes as scholars and human beings have been affected by their experiences as qualitative organizational researchers). I have attempted to illustrate some of these processes by relating the experiences of six organizational researchers who have spent the bulk of their careers carrying out qualitative research. Three of these scholars are senior faculty: Bob Sutton, Stanford University; Kathy Eisenhardt, Stanford University; and Steve Barley, Stanford University. The other three are junior faculty: C. V. Harquail, University of Virginia; Mike Pratt, University of Illinois; and Mark Zbaracki, University of Chicago. I asked these scholars to describe the process of becoming and remaining a qualitative researcher and how that process has had real effects on their personal and professional identities.

Before I relate these stories, however, I will provide a brief overview of the types of qualitative research these scholars have carried out. I will also comment on the literature, to date, that has examined the experiences of qualitative researchers in organizational studies.

QUALITATIVE FIELD RESEARCH IN ORGANIZATIONS

Qualitative research in organizational settings (e.g., private and public corporations and businesses, government organizations, and special interest associations) falls, roughly, into two major categories: (a) single instrumental case studies involving long-term participant observation or ethnography in a single research site and (b) collective instrumental case studies involving interviews and nonparticipant observation across several research sites (Stake, 1994). In both of these methods, the organizational researcher is searching for insight about a specific phenomenon.[1] The level of analysis in these case studies may be the individual, group, or organization level, and the researchers' level of interaction with the research context may range from distanced observer to full participant. A brief illustration of these forms of inquiry follows.

Single Case Studies

Typically, single case studies involve an in-depth and long-term analysis of the lives of organization members. Furthermore, these studies often focus on unusual or extreme examples of a phenomenon as means of illustrating its full range of manifestations. For example, the authors interviewed for this chapter have published the following papers based on single, in-depth case studies:

"The Happiest, Most Dissatisfied People on Earth: Ambivalence and Commitment Among Amway Distributors" (Pratt, 1994)
"Navigating by Attire: The Use of Dress by Female Administrative Employees" (Rafaeli, Dutton, Harquail, & Mackie-Lewis, 1997)
"Maintaining Organizational Norms About Expressed Emotions: The Case of Bill Collectors" (Sutton, 1991)

"Brainstorming Groups in Context: Effectiveness in a Product Design Firm" (Sutton & Hargadon, 1996)

"Untangling the Relationship Between Displayed Emotions and Organizational Sales: The Case of Convenience Stores" (Sutton & Rafaeli, 1988)

"Client Disclosure and Demeanor as Sources of Enjoyment for Hair Stylists: An Ethnographic Study" (Sutton & Cohen, 1994).

Qualitative researchers using this method often become at least partial participants in the research context and refer to themselves as *ethnographers* to differentiate themselves from less involved case study researchers who rely primarily on interviews or nonparticipant observation. As a result, it seems probable that such researchers would have experiences that profoundly affect their personal and professional identities.

Collective Case Studies

In contrast to single case studies, collective case studies typically involve nonparticipant observation and post-hoc interviews with organization members about events that occurred in the recent past. These methods are more efficient and easier to standardize for researchers who wish to compare and contrast findings across multiple research sites. Although such methods are more removed from the research context than are ethnographic methods, the quantity of information uncovered and the range of people interviewed may have a strong, cumulative effect on the researcher that equals the impact of more in-depth methods. Recent examples of this methodology, used by authors interviewed for this paper, include:

"Technology as an Occasion for Structuring: Evidence From Observations of CT Scanners and the Social Order of Radiology Departments" (Barley, 1986)

"Technicians in the Workplace: Ethnographic Evidence for Bringing Work Into Organization Studies" (Barley, 1996)

"Strategic Decision Processes in High Velocity Environments: Four Cases in the Microcomputer Industry" (Bourgeois & Eisenhardt, 1988)

"The Art of Continuous Change: Linking Complexity Theory and Time-Paced Revolution in Relentlessly Shifting Organizations" (Brown & Eisenhardt, 1997)

"What People Say and What People Do: The Rhetoric and Reality of Change" (Zbaracki, 1998)

Although long-term ethnography at a single research site has a distinguished history in the social sciences (see Vidich and Lyman, 1994, for a review) and has been used since the earliest qualitative studies of organizations (Becker, Greer, Hughes, & Strauss, 1961), multiple case studies appear to be growing in popularity in current organizational literature. This may be due, in part, to the greater perceived generalizability and reliability of findings that are based on multiple cases versus a single case and to the publication of methodological reviews in organizational journals that help to standardize and legitimate the multiple-case-method form (Eisenhardt, 1989).

LITERATURE ON THE EXPERIENCES OF QUALITATIVE ORGANIZATIONAL RESEARCHERS

Although the foregoing discussion suggests that qualitative organizational researchers are involved in research contexts that should have profound effects on how they see themselves and their world, commentary on such effects is relatively rare among organizational researchers. Only a handful of insightful articles have been written about the personal experiences of organizational qualitative researchers, including discussions of so-called "impressionist ethnography" (Van Maanen, 1988), of case studies of emotionally hot topics (Sutton & Schurman, 1985), and what's known as "action research" (Coghlan, 1994). These writings appear to confirm the notion that qualitative organizational researchers are aware of their place in the research experience. Yet this awareness is focused on how their personal biases and subjective interpretations of data affect the theory that results from their studies. Much less is said about the effects of the research experience on their professional or personal identities.

Impressionist Ethnography

Van Maanen (1988) defines a form of ethnography that is composed of a series of remembered events in which the author-participant chooses to reconstruct only those events he or she regards as especially notable and reportable as *impressionist tales*. According to Van Maanen, these tales are affected by the researcher's participation in the research context because the researcher him or herself is affected by this experience. In fact, it is the researcher's subjective impression of the research scene, based on his or her engagement in that scene, that is the focus of this form of ethnography. Relating and recreating this experience is the means by which the researcher communicates with his or her audience. As Van Maanen notes,

> The audience is asked to relive the tale with the fieldworker, not interpret or analyze it. The intention is not to tell readers what to think of an experience but to show them the experience from beginning to end and thus draw them immediately into the story to work out its problems and puzzles as they unfold. . . . Fieldworkers, as impressionists, take some pride in demonstrating that they were anything but simple scribes, absorbent sponges, or academic ciphers in their research

worlds. Such disinterested characters would hardly make engaging narrators for an impressionist tale. (pp. 103, 104)

Van Maanen (1988) illustrates this form of qualitative research by relating his own experience in a study of police officers. In this impressionist tale, he describes not only what the cops appear to be feeling and thinking during the apprehension of a car thief but what he is feeling and thinking as a participant in the action. In describing this experience later, he suggests that it changed his perceptions not only of police officers but of himself. For instance,

> What I learned from this little episode and its many tellings is that I wasn't as smart or as detached in the field as I thought I was and had, in fact, presented myself as being in my confessional writings. I was frightened but thrilled by the chase, touched by guilt because I was so fearful and slow to emerge from the prowl car after the crash, maddened by my inability to operate the machinery or find my way around an area I had spent considerable time in, frustrated yet crazed with the idea of capturing the little car thief, puzzled by the confusion on the scene, surprised by the actions (or inactions) of both myself and some of my colleagues, and, in general, somewhat ashamed but mostly amused by the buffoonery of the night shift. (p. 116)

In particular, the foregoing passage indicates that qualitative researchers may become increasingly introspective, becoming more and more aware of their shortcomings and strengths, through multiple retellings of their research experiences. In this respect, it appears that doing impressionist qualitative ethnography may affect one's professional and personal identity.

Case Studies of Emotionally Hot Topics

Sutton and Schurman (1985) discuss the researcher experience in qualitative case studies of emotionally hot topics in organizations. They describe the emotional demands and coping strategies researchers may experience in studying organizational death (e.g., the closing of a business). Their discussion reveals that qualitative scholars' close relationship with their informants may have a strong impact on their self-perceptions as researchers. Specifically, Sutton and Schurman note that in studying plant closings, upset informants expected more from researchers than do informants in less emotional settings:

> They often expect the researcher to abandon the traditional, emotionally neutral posture and adopt a more clinical posture.... They expected us to listen attentively when they discussed personal problems. . . . Informants often asked us, "what did managers in other closings do in this situation?" . . . Many informants insisted that they had better get plenty of feedback about our findings. (p. 339)

In response to these demands, the researchers found themselves taking on the role of therapist with many informants. Furthermore, this role was adhered to even when the emotions of the research context began to affect the researchers' own well-being.

> At times, we would have to work very hard not to lose our tempers at informants who attacked us personally. . . . Guilt was also a common response among those of us on the research team. We worried that the fellow who accused social scientists of voyeurism was correct. . . . The distress evoked within us by these emotional episodes sometimes interfered with our performance on subsequent research tasks. Some members of the research team responded to their own guilt and anger with psychological detachment from informants and procrastination. . . . Clearly, not performing research tasks interferes with the quality of the research. But psychological and behavioral detachment are not without virtue. These "time-outs" helped us to continue our long-term efforts. Despite the widely advertised evils of procrastination, putting off phone calls for a few weeks *helped us regain our ability to be supportive* [italics added] and reduced the probability that we would abandon the research. (Sutton & Schurman, 1985, p. 340)

This passage indicates that the demands of research informants changed, at least temporally, the professional identities of researchers from detached scientists to concerned friends or counselors.

Action Research

Last, organizational action research methodologies also require the researcher to become involved in the organizational context he or she is studying (Argyris, Putnam, & Smith, 1985; Lewin, 1973). Coghlan (1994) summarizes the concept of action research as follows:

> It involves change experiments on real problems in social systems. . . . It, like social management more generally, involves iterative cycles of identifying a problem, planning, acting, and evaluating. . . . The intended change in an action research project typically involves re-education, a term that refers to changing patterns of thinking and action that are presently well-established in individuals and groups. . . . *It challenges the status quo from a participative perspective, which is congruent with the requirements of effective re-education* [italics added]. (p. 120)

Researchers using this method of inquiry have written, briefly, about the importance of recognizing the subjective nature of one's observations and of the influence of one's participation in the research experience. In this vein, Carl Rogers (as cited in Coghlan, 1994) defines the concept of *in-dwelling* as a method "whereby the scientist develops a mode experience of empathy with the perceptions/attitudes/feelings/behavior or experience of the client-participant" (p. 125). Similarly, Schein (1987) describes the action researchers role as "clinical," because it puts the scientist in the position of an expert helper, who diagnoses an organizational context based on his or her participation in the research context.

Yet Mirvis and Seashore (1982) note that this experience may also have some unintended and negative consequences for the researcher. In particular, they warn that, because action researchers are asked to intervene and change a system but also become participants in the research context, they may have difficulty making decisions that place organizational needs counter to employee needs. For example, it may be difficult for an empathetic researcher to suggest downsizing a department in which he or she has become an insider. In confronting such dilemmas, the action researcher is likely to discover or affirm something about his or her professional identity, as well as his or her personal character. Thus, similar to the earlier discussion of emotionally hot topics, research in action domains places the researcher in an unconventional relationship with his or her subjects (i.e., as a therapist or clinician). In turn, such relationships seem likely to affect the self-perceptions and social identities of scholars in unconventional ways.

SIX STORIES OF
RESEARCHER EXPERIENCE

Although the foregoing review suggests that qualitative researchers may be aware of how their experiences in the field have affected them, discourse on this topic is fairly thin and focuses on how researcher experiences affect the output of their studies (e.g., the quality of theory or insights), rather than how such experiences affect the researchers themselves (e.g., their self-perceptions or identities). To provide a starting point for thinking about how the identities of qualitative organizational researchers have been affected by their experiences in the field, I conducted semistructured interviews with the six scholars introduced at the beginning of the chapter (Bob Sutton, Kathy Eisenhardt, Steve Barley, C. V. Harquail, Mike Pratt, and Mark Zbaracki). These interviews were not meant to provide a formal framework about the experience of being a qualitative researcher but instead, to serve as a catalyst for conversation and thinking about how doing qualitative organizational research affects the identities of the researcher.

I have organized these stories into sets of insights produced by each of the informants. Each insight is summarized by an opening quote and then explained in more detail through interview text. I report only those insights that the researchers themselves indicated were important moments for them as qualitative organizational theorists.

Bob Sutton

The longer I do research, the more I realize that, in some ways, the quantity of data I have is really incredibly unrelated to how good a story I can tell.

One of the most profound things that happened to me was when I read this book *Termination: The Closing of the Baker Plant.* This is a book written by a journalist and it is the only piece of nonfiction he ever wrote. It's about a plant closing in Detroit in the 1960s. A plant closing, by the way, which was the subject of extensive quantitative research. His name is Al Slote. I talked to him, really sweet guy. You can tell that he did these interviews, but he just kept rough notes. He's a professional novelist. He wrote murder mysteries that were set in the Michigan Law School, called the *Santa Claus Capers.* The dialogue of this *Termination* book is too good. But in many ways, my dissertation is just a formalization of his whole book. There are a few pages of this book that are about the part where they got drunk and recalled the place for themselves. Reading that passage was an inspiration that led to a whole paper and a focus that I had on dying organizations.

My first reason for doing research in general is as an excuse to interact with people I like, and my second reason is to get stuff done.

If I get enough stuff done, then I'm fine with that. But the other side of it is incredibly unproductive. So in this paper at [a design firm], you might be able to see the multiple motivations I had for doing the study, many of which were quite impure. One is that I wanted to spend time hanging out with Joe [a senior manager] because he's a nice guy, and I wanted to get to know him better, so that was relatively pure. But let's look at the impure motivations. One is that I wanted to remain in the good graces of Rick and Joe [the firm's top managers], and this is the kind of thing that meant a lot to Joe. But, I've become such an insider there that I don't know whether I can be objective at all about anything anymore. I'm such a player in the system that, politically, I have an agenda, I have people I'm aligned with, I have people I'm not aligned with. Luckily, I'm aligned with the CEO and his brother who run the company and the CEO of its partner company. So I'm clearly viewed as in a top management coalition, and the only people who will trust me beyond that, on certain levels, are people who've known me forever, including a lot of former Stanford students. So in that case, it's been totally warped to the point where I've become an insider and I'm not objective at all.

C. V. Harquail

It's so important when you're there to identify and be empathic and let the people tell you their story. But at the same time, it really hurts.

When I was interviewing the women in the ad agency about their advocacy efforts on behalf of women, some of them told me stories that just broke my heart. Sometimes, it was hard not to start crying in the interview. And to remain empathic and open and listening while the whole time you're like, "oh my God, what an awful story." And then you go back and you listen to the tapes again or the transcription comes back from the secretary and you just read it and think "it's hard feeling other people's pain." I would often do two interviews and then be so glad I couldn't have a third one scheduled that day because I just needed to go have a cup of coffee. And I spent a lot of time writing in my journal, especially with my dissertation study, because these women were doing jobs that I could really see myself doing. And they were in situations where their values or identities were challenged, situations that I could really imagine myself being in. And some of them copped out and didn't advocate for women's issues, they just didn't step up to the plate. And others did. And I often asked myself, "well, what would I have done?" Would I have been the person who just said, "I'm going to keep my nose clean and I'm going to get promoted" or would I have stuck up for somebody? So I identified in some sense with these women.

I had to quickly decide if I was going to present myself as fairly much the opposite of who I was. Not like an ardent right-winger, but somewhere sort of on the other side of the dimension.

Here's another identification dilemma that I had in this study. Most of the time, although I'm toned down a lot, it's pretty clear I'm a feminist. It's probably pretty clear I'm a Democrat. It's pretty clear I'm liberal. All those sorts of things. And that worked fine when I would get into an interview and discover that the woman who I was interviewing in fact identified with women as a group and in fact was aware of sexism or discrimination and was making small efforts to do something about it. That worked fine because I didn't have to change who I was in order to connect with her. But I always had to kind of hold back who I was until I found out who she was. And that wasn't terribly much of a problem until I walked into one woman's office and I sat down and looked behind her and on her bulletin board she had this framed picture of herself being hugged by Ronald Reagan. I said, "Wow, you know Ronald Reagan" and I was going to say, "Ew, how could you let him hug you?" or something like that. And I realized that I had just sat down in the office of Phyllis Schaffley's disciple. This woman was hyper right wing and the absolute opposite of me. . . . So I held back many of my more liberal opinions in that interview.

I really had to ask myself, "Is this my agenda or is this real?"

In the dress study, Anat and Jane were the principal investigators and early in our data analysis discussions, Anat and I were on very opposite sides about whether this whole dress at work thing was an issue that was specifically important to women, or more important to women than men. I was completely convinced that dress was much more complex for women because of the different stereotypes they have to handle and the different kind of role conflicts they encounter. We just happened to be interviewing women because we wanted to look at administrators and they were all women. And Anat was like no, no, no, the "women" thing is not that big a thing. And, as it ended up, the line of analysis about women and dress became more prominent, and became one of the arguments that we made. But it didn't come as strongly and with the same kind of emphasis as it would have if I had written the paper by myself. I think it was really funny because I was sure that that was in the data, and Anat was sure that it wasn't, so every time I would point out where it was, she would say, "no, it's really not there." Since she was teaching me how to do qualitative data analysis, I had to keep reconsidering, "well, maybe it's not there."

I felt at that point that my responsibility had shifted from gathering data about this woman's experience, to "I have something I can share with her that is going to make a difference."

I had one interview with a woman who was talking about a friend at work who had breast cancer and how she filled in for her and she did things like tell other people about how her friend's chemo was going, and all this kind of stuff, really trying to be a bridge between that woman's coping with the disease and her work life. As it happened, when I was doing my dissertation, one of my very best friends at grad school was dying of breast cancer. So although I knew it when it was happening, I kind of veered off my interview protocol, and we really had a heart-to-heart talk about what it took to support somebody who was facing breast cancer. And that was really weird because I knew when I was shifting gears in our conversation that I was violating all sorts of things I had been taught about objectivity.

Even though I know in general I'm quick to judge, I really think that I have become much more open-minded and much more willing to have conversations with people with whom I don't agree, instead of having combative conversations with them.

I'm much more willing to ask people "why do you think that way?" or "that kind of surprises me, I wouldn't have thought that, can you tell me more?" And with research participants, I want to leave them feeling like they've learned something about themselves and that the interview has been interesting. You know, as if they bumped into somebody on an airplane and had so much fun talking to the person about something they usually didn't think about that they end up forgetting that the flight was delayed by an hour and a half. So I think now I can have conversations with just about anyone.

Mike Pratt

Once I did [qualitative research], it was one of those things where it became very difficult to go back to the survey research stuff because the qualitative research was so invigorating. It really was renewing for me. It got me excited about the kind of stuff that I was doing.

> For me, qualitative research is pretty much up front. It has its flaws, but they hang out there. We don't say it's one thing and it's actually something else. And I like that about it. I think it was affirming of my identity in a couple of different ways. First, I thought it was intellectually more honest. It also fits more with how I believe the world is. That is, as researchers, we don't necessarily know more about an organization than the people in the organization do. We may have different kinds of knowledge, but I've always felt that people who are out there in the trenches really know a lot more about what's going on than we do as researchers. It's our responsibility to find out what they know, not to see how they conform to our theories.

I've always felt like an outlier in the business school.

> I mean, and I went into psychology as a grad student. At the time, I swore I would never be in a business school because I was in psychology and I was there to help people, that kind of stuff. So I really resonated with qualitative research because I felt I wasn't just doing research, but I could really help in the grander scheme of things. There are times when that gets kind of frustrating, though. I think that the choice of being a qualitative researcher can alienate you from other academics. If you're branded as a qualitative researcher, you may be perceived as having less to talk about with other colleagues because the methodology gets in the way.

The Amway study has changed me. I talk about the one study that has changed the way I look at the world, that would be it.

> First of all, it kind of made me realize the power of giving people hope at kind of a basic level. Also, in learning how Amway was really successful, I became interested in ambivalence and the process of making people incredibly uncomfortable or ambivalent about their lives. "This is who you want to be, this is who you are now, can you see that it's not the same. If you don't go for it, then you're a loser." I remember giving this talk and saying, okay, what would you do to get tenure? Would you work extra hours, work really late at night to get something published, would you work weekends? Then it started to click. Oh. . . .Yeah, we're doing exactly the same thing in academia as Amway does with its members. And I had actually a whole chapter in my dissertation about the similarities between graduate school and Amway training and this kind of combination

of making people really uncomfortable with who they are, never being satisfied with what you have right now. I look at someone like Karl Weick, who I had a class with, and he said, you know, I still don't know if I've made it, or I still don't think I'm as smart as people think I am. I said wow, if someone like Karl can be at that point, what are we creating as a profession. These people are constantly dissatisfied with who they are. The title of my dissertation was "The Happiest Most Dissatisfied People on Earth." In some ways, you feel a sense of accomplishment about what you're doing, but it's not happiness, there's no contentment there.

In terms of research, [the Amway study] probably made me more committed than ever to qualitative methods. I would never have been able to understand what Amway people really are going through if I hadn't done it myself.

The ethnography honed in this feeling even more. I felt I had tapped into some really fundamental organizational dynamics that I had not experienced before; identity transformation, how organizations change who we are and how we think about ourselves. It was interesting because, before I did the Amway study, I wrote what I called a "time capsule," saying this is where I'm at in my life at this point. I didn't read it until I was done with the project, to see if I had changed. It was funny. I don't know if I had changed that much, but just to kind of see where I was, what my concerns were before the study, and going back to it a year later, it was really kind of neat.

Also, it's probably the most difficult project I've done in the sense that one thing I'd found out is, I couldn't live my life as an academic and be in Amway at the same time.

To be in Amway and really have the courage to let go of my academic identity was hard. There were a couple jokes that I didn't quite take as jokes. They would say "Oh, are you converted yet?" or somebody else said, "You're starting to use the term *we* now." But to be an academic, you constantly have to be very skeptical, which doesn't fit with being an Amway member. In Amway, you can't be skeptical or you can't be in that community. Going back and forth was so psychologically stressful and draining that at one point, I just told my committee, "I'll talk to you in 5 or 6 months about this. If you see me, I don't want to talk about Amway." I really got immersed, and I could tell in my research journal, because I kept fairly extensive research notes, at some point saying, you know, I know I shouldn't really believe this stuff, but it's all starting to make sense. From the inside, it made a tremendous amount of sense; as an academic, it looked incredibly absurd.

I was really worried that somebody had basically taken what I read and said, "You know, you make me look like I'm some kind of sleazeball."

Amway had sponsored me, and they had done a lot of work to help me with the project, so I gave them a special bound copy of it. Before they read it, they gave it to their up-line to read, to make sure they were basically okay with that. The way Amway works, you can't have negative thoughts. So they wanted to make sure that it was okay to read. I keep thinking they were like "thought police" and stuff like that, but that's probably a little bit overboard. And then one distributor told me he didn't like it at all, because it made him feel like he was a huckster. I felt that I had gone out of my way to display both good and bad. And by contrast, most people would have written a scathing expose. But I said no, but there are some really good things about Amway that I want to include. And for him not to realize that I had tried to do that hurt a lot. I actually asked another Amway distributor who wasn't in the book to read it. And, to my relief, he said, "You know, not everything is exactly what I had experienced, but this is a really fair treatment of it." He said, "You've pretty much got it on track." And that made me feel a lot better.

You're almost like an ambassador. Because if you make the wrong translation between party A and party B, you can start a war, or you could cause a lot of harm to either side.

I think, as a qualitative researcher, if you're trying to reflect what people within the context are thinking and how they're doing things, you have more responsibility to make sure you do things right. Because a lot of people only know Amway through talks. If you give a very negative view of this organization, you have much more of a responsibility to make sure you do things accurately. I think that was part of the reason why it was difficult to write the Amway stuff, because I felt I needed to include enough positive information to prevent people from forming a jaded or narrow view of the organization. I thought, unless I have balanced story here, I can't publish it, because it's not fair to the people who I work with. So that was a good reminder for me of the responsibility qualitative researchers have.

Steve Barley

I know what I believe, and I know what I do, and I know that what I do gets published, and I don't have to run around whining about why my work's not getting done.

My identity is as a realist ethnographer. Which is not to say that I don't buy the social construction argument. It's just that I'm a realist ethnographer. I believe there is a reality that is socially constructed, but it's real. As real as anything else. So I'm not into peeling back layer after layer of the onion. I really don't have a lot of patience for research that does that. But I also don't want to be involved in these arguments, either. That's the other thing I've learned over the years. I want to steer clear of these arguments about what constitutes righteous qualitative research.

I hate the minutia of doing a quantitative analysis. I just hate it.

And what I hate even worse is finding that you made this little teeny, fucking mistake somewhere, and you got all the way down to the point where you're about to write something, and you go, "Oh, God damn. You know, my coefficient was screwed up or I multiplied this wrong," or "Oh shit, this was a singular matrix." God, I hate that.

I think that people can tell you a lot of things, but I think that if you really want to know what people think, you have to look at what they do rather than what they say.

What I learned in my CT scanner study was how to do observation in ways that were potentially countable. I really became an ethnographer who focuses on behaviors. So if you look closely at my work, I'm always talking as much about what people do as what they say, and often my work focuses more on what people do than what they say. And even when they say things, I'm interested in how they say things and under what situations. So I don't use much interview data. If I'm in a situation long enough, I don't need to interview anybody.

All my work, for the most part, has been driven by my own interest in social issues. It has to do with why I personally choose problems in the first place.

I think it's easier to understand the dynamics of certain kinds of social problems from a qualitative perspective, and that's what I like about doing my research. And I've certainly been exposed to lots of things that quantitative researchers don't get exposed to because they're not that close to the people they're actually writing about or the scenes they're actually writing about. For example, I think I have a better appreciation for the fundamental nobility of work, regardless of how simple it seems. It's far more complex than it appears on the surface.

Kathy Eisenhardt

I think qualitative research makes you theoretically sharper as well as being more applied.

I don't think I've ever done a study that had no qualitative data in it. Why? Because not only do you learn what the critical variables are and how they affect each other, but you've been there and observed the phenomenon. You speak about it more as an insider rather than just as a person who has minimal understanding. I think qualitative data make me theoretically much better. Because, for me, understanding a phenomenon qualitatively is not about "therefore, you can be more applied." It's about, "therefore, you're more likely to have an accurate theoretical understanding." So, it's really that the insight is more valid.

The impact of qualitative data was just huge. And if all we'd done was measure it, if all we'd done was questionnaires, we never would have seen it. It was all in the qualitative data.

We were doing a study of politics. That was what we planned to do. And when we got to talking with the executives at the companies, the only thing they wanted to talk about was speed. It was all about speed. All about pace. And in retrospect, it seems hard to believe that we wouldn't have known that that was what was going to happen. But we didn't. And in the end, issues related to speed have become the enduring theme of my career for the past 10 years or so—speed and competition and fast-paced industries.

I think one of the things that qualitative data has made me appreciate is how hard a lot of people work, and how tough it is in business today, and how rhetoric about the self-interest of managers is really missing the point for most managers.

Most managers that I see work extremely hard, are very concerned about the people who work for them, and are just overall trying to do a good job in a very difficult situation, a very competitive situation, a place that most of us in academics probably wouldn't want to be. I don't know how many times I've heard people say to me, "If I had to do this career over again, I would never get in this business. This business is a killer business." I think I've increasingly been sympathetic to how tough it is and how people are trying, not to rip off their customers, but to do the right thing, and it's hard to manage well when it's so competitive.

Sometimes, I think that managers believe that I've said, "Tell me about what you're doing here, and by the way, you can complain because I'm not going to tell anybody you said it."

I'm not one of them, and I don't do the ethnographies that other people do. Rather, I do more "go in for a few hours and talk to some people." I interview one person for a few hours and then talk to somebody else. I hang around for a while. But I don't hang there for a long time. This lets me see more variety. But it also makes me like a therapist. I guess the closest role is probably a shrink. And I know that managers tell us much more than they planned to.

Mark Zbaracki

And in some senses, in retrospect, the technical stuff that I was studying was less interesting to me than simply finding out about their lives and kind of what they were up to.

I enjoyed meeting the different people, seeing what they were up to, looking at the different contexts in which they were working, finding out what their lives were about. It's just fascinating to me to see them in their work settings, hear them talk about their backgrounds, describe what it was that they were doing. I could hear themes of my own background echoing, and I liked that. You know, here was something in common. I could look at the tensions and kind of try to understand where they were coming from. I could look at what they thought was really cool and see that. I could look at their backgrounds. I keep remembering, at the Sacramento site, there were all these folks from the same church. And so one of the things that was sort of puzzling to me was the number of these people from that church running around the organization, and why was it? Why were they hiring so many people from that church? How did that affect what it was that they were up to? You know, here I am studying technology, but to me what's more interesting is their kind of background. What do they do with the rest of their lives? How does it affect what they do there?

I come out of a background in engineering, and my entire life, there's been this tension between an interest in engineering and an interest in the humanities.

When I was an undergraduate, I would take humanities courses on the side. They sort of got me through the engineering work. And so there was this abiding interest that was kind of suppressed for years and for years and for years and for years. And here I am in an engineering kind of program but with this other interest that just keeps popping up. And you know, it was almost an irrepressible side of myself. It just wasn't interesting to me to think about running huge data sets. It still isn't. You know, it drives me nuts when people get off into arcane data issues. I keep saying there's a story there, and I'm more interested in the story than I am in the data. And so, this is sort of like my true identity that's been suppressed for all these years. And in some senses, it would never have occurred to me to go do a lab experiment, but it was way more interesting for me to get into people stories. What do they have to say about their lives? I mean, it's a theme that becomes increasingly strong as I look at what it is that I'm doing. But I look back to my images of doing that kind of stuff, and the technical stuff, particularly on that project, wasn't terribly interesting to me. But meeting the people was a lot of fun. So I used to look forward to the trips to these different sites. You know, the notion of getting in my car and driving several hours, spending the night there. I was going to get up the next morning and meet all these different folks. That I really liked. But it was also that I felt an affinity for these people. You know, I had seen those kinds of problems, and I could identify with what it was that they were saying. So, in terms of identity, it wasn't so much that my choice was necessarily better, because there were different dimensions to my choices in academia that were problematic for me. It was that, yeah, I understood what it was that they were doing. And I guess I kind of admired them for their commitment to what it was that they were doing, in that context.

I learned that people don't want to know the truth all the time. And I haven't yet resolved that issue as a qualitative scholar.

If you remember, the first site that I studied, they wanted some overview when all was said and done. And so, in coming up with the overview, I told them, here's what I see. And it wasn't the story they particularly wanted to hear. I mean, there were some folks in there, lower in the organization, who certainly wanted to hear this, but the people higher up in the organization didn't hear what it was that I wanted to say. And so they never talked to me again. Once that happened, it was pretty clear I was no longer wanted around that organization. Bob always says that in the end, you always turn on your informants. Well, I did it in a hurry at that particular site.

That's sort of where I get frustrated with academia in general, is that we're not necessarily experts.

Where I get really exasperated with business schools in general is that somehow, we want to pass ourselves off as experts, and my perception of the world is that it's way more mysterious than we can possibly imagine. It's just way more complicated. And so, certainly over the past few years, I've been increasingly aware of how important people's stories are to them. How unimportant theory, ultimately, is to them. How important it is for them to do well. And how frankly powerless we are to help them.

CONCLUSION

The six stories I've just reported appear to confirm the notion that understanding how qualitative researchers have been personally affected by their experiences in real-life organizations should help them and others understand how their data and its interpretation may be intertwined with their own values and beliefs. At a minimum, a realization of the extent to which qualitative researchers are, in fact, genuinely affected by their research experiences should help others to *experience* the findings of qualitative studies and to interpret those findings within that experience—much as the original researcher had. Yet these stories go beyond that notion by suggesting that, in addition to affecting perceptions of their work, the experiences of qualitative organizational researchers may also affect perceptions of themselves. That is, the foregoing stories suggest that doing qualitative research may change our identities as scholars and human beings.

As scholars, doing qualitative research may change our identities in terms of the kinds of issues we find interesting, the kinds of theories we find useful, and the kinds of insights we find important to pass on to students and colleagues. As human beings, doing qualitative research may change our identities by debunking stereotypes and improving our ability to take another's perspective. In general, an informal analysis of the insights reported in this paper suggests three broad categories of insights that may affect the personal and professional identities of qualitative organizational researchers: (a) insights about one's relationship with informants, (b) insights about one's personal and professional growth, and (c) insights about affirming one's self-perception as unconventional. These insights are summarized in Table 6.1.

First, it was clear to me that all of the qualitative researchers interviewed for this chapter had experiences with their informants that changed their views of their role as researcher and, in some cases, their identification with stereotypical views of organizational theorists. Some researchers felt a responsibility to act as a therapist or counselor, whereas others felt they should at least be empathetic and act as ambassadors in relating informants' stories to the public. A couple mentioned the importance of suppressing personal opinions and beliefs that conflicted with those of their informants to make those informants feel more comfortable. These are not identities these researchers anticipated when entering their academic careers. Yet most of them admitted enjoying the new relationships with informants and found them a important motivator for continuing qualitative research. Furthermore, a couple of the researchers noted that working at these relationships helped their communication skills and relationships outside of their professional roles. Apparently, the difficult task of confronting their informants with negative results made these researchers more sensitive to how they presented criticism to others. Qualitative researchers, it appears, often become better listeners and conversationalists through their interactions with informants.

In a related vein, a number of researchers claimed to have matured as scholars and people. Most claimed to have a greater appreciation for the workers they observed, as well as for the effectiveness of qualitative methods for uncovering theoretical insights. Some also claimed to have become more accepting of their identities as qualitative researchers, even if that identity was not valued by many of their colleagues. This acceptance appeared to come from appreciating the importance of their informants' stories for the advancement of theory and the improvement of management practices.

Table 6.1 Being a Qualitative, Organizational Researcher: Insights and Self-Perceptions

Professional Insights *Relationship With Informants*	**Personal Insights** *Relationship With Informants*
It's important to identify and empathize in doing qualitative research. Qualitative research can present the identity dilemma of having to show a false self-image to informants. Qualitative researchers have a great responsibility to their subjects to act as ambassadors to the public. Qualitative researchers may find themselves in the role of therapist to subjects.	A primary motivation for doing qualitative research is talking to or observing people. Qualitative research sometimes presents opportunities for helping informants outside of the research goals. Qualitative researchers often must face negative, hurtful reactions from their subjects. Qualitative research may reveal truths people don't want to hear.
Professional Growth	*Personal Growth*
Quantity of data is unrelated to quality of story. Interpreting qualitative data can be heavily influenced by one's own research agendas. Doing qualitative research can bring an awareness of phenomena not visible through any other method. Qualitative research can make a person theoretically sharper and more accurate. Qualitative research can heighten appreciation about how little scholars really know about organizations.	Doing qualitative research can make one more open-minded. Qualitative research can profoundly change one's view of the world. Qualitative researchers are often driven by their personal interests in social issues. Qualitative research can debunk stereotypes of organizations and their members.
Affirming Unconventional Identities	*Affirming Unconventional Identities*
Doing qualitative research allows one to maintain the identity of an "outsider" in a business school. Qualitative researchers must be self-accepting in their professional identities, even if they're not accepted by others.	Qualitative research fits a personality style that is more experiential and hands-on. Qualitative research is a way of balancing personal tensions between quantitative and qualitative interests.

Last, most of the researchers interviewed claimed that doing qualitative research enabled them, in some way, to affirm their identities as unconventional people. For example, a couple noted that they could not identify with the stereotype of a business school professor and felt their research methods allowed them to separate themselves from that stereotype. Others indicated that they disidentified with quantitative methods because of early experiences as doctoral students, in which they came to find those methods uninspiring. Still others suggested that they thought of themselves as rebellious and independent in general, and this was just one more way of affirming that part of their identities.

In sum, this chapter suggests that the experiences of qualitative organizational researchers may lead those researchers to see themselves as more adept communicators, mature scholars, and unconventional individuals in comparison to their quantitative counterparts. They certainly see themselves as thinking differently than quantitative researchers. Although these notions are based on a limited set of interviews, they ring true for my own experiences with qualitative researchers over the past 10 years. Although my data is far too preliminary to comment on the potential consequences of these findings, it seems clear that the identity differences between qualitative and quantitative researchers may have shaped the nature of discourse in organizational studies and may continue to have a profound impact on the development of paradigms in this field as this method becomes increasingly popular.

NOTE

1. By contrast, sociological researchers using what is called *intrinsic case study* are looking to better understand a particular research site, with no predefined agenda for examining specific events or phenomena. This type of qualitative research is relatively rare in organizational studies, and I will not focus on it in this chapter.

REFERENCES

Argyris, C., Putnam, R., & Smith, D. (1985). *Action science.* San Francisco: Jossey-Bass.

Barley, S. R. (1986). Technology as an occasion for structuring: Evidence from observations of CT scanners and the social order of radiology departments. *Administrative Science Quarterly, 31,* 78-108.

Barley, S. R. (1996). Technicians in the workplace: Ethnographic evidence for bringing work into organization studies. *Administrative Science Quarterly, 41,* 404-441.

Becker, H. S., Greer, B., Hughes, E. C., & Strauss, A. L. (1961). *Boys in white: Student culture in medical school.* Chicago: University of Chicago Press.

Bourgeois, L. J., & Eisenhardt, K. (1988). Strategic decision processes in high velocity environments: Four cases in the microcomputer industry. *Management Science, 34,* 816-835.

Brown, S. L., & Eisenhardt, K. M. (1997). The art of continuous change: Linking complexity theory and time-paced evolution in relentlessly shifting organizations. *Administrative Science Quarterly, 42,* 1-34.

Coghlan, D. (1994). Research as a process of change: Action science in organisations. *Irish Business & Administrative Research, 15,* 119-30.

Eisenhardt, K. M. (1989). Making fast strategic decisions in high-velocity environments. *Academy of Management Journal, 32,*543-576.

Lewin, K. (1973). Action research and minority problems. In K. Lewin (Ed.), *Resolving social conflicts: Selected papers in group dynamics.* London: Souvenir Press.

Mirvis, P. H., & Seashore, S. E. (1982). Being ethical in organizational research. In J. Seiber (Ed.), *The ethics of social research.* New York: Springer-Verlag.

Pratt, M. G. (1994). *The happiest, most dissatisfied people on earth: Ambivalence and commitment among Amway distributors.* Unpublished dissertation, University of Michigan, Ann Arbor.

Rafaeli, A., Dutton, J., Harquail, C. V., & Mackie-Lewis, S. (1997). Navigating by attire: The use of dress by female administrative employees. *Academy of Management Journal, 40,* 9-45.

Schein, E. H. (1987). *The clinical perspective in fieldwork.* Newbury Park, CA: Sage.

Schlenker, B. R. (1986). Self-identification: Toward an integration of the private and public self. In R. F. Baumister (Ed.), *Public self and private self* (pp. 21-62). New York: Springer-Verlag.

Stake, R. E. (1994). Case studies. In N. K. Denzin & Y. S. Lincoln (Eds.), *Handbook of qualitative research* (pp. 236-247). Thousand Oaks, CA: Sage.

Sutton, R. I. (1991). Maintaining organizational norms about expressed emotions: The case of bill collectors. *Administrative Science Quarterly, 36,* 245-268.

Sutton, R. I., & Cohen, R. C. (1994, August). *Client disclosure and demeanor as sources of enjoyment for hair stylists: An ethnographic study.* Paper presented at the annual meetings of the Academy of Management, Dallas, Texas.

Sutton, R. I., & Hargadon, A. (1996). Brainstorming groups in context: Effectiveness in a product design firm. *Administrative Science Quarterly, 41,* 685-718.

Sutton, R. I., & Rafaeli, A. (1988). Untangling the relationship between displayed emotions and organizational sales: The case of convenience stores. *Academy of Management Journal, 31,* 461-487.

Sutton, R. I., & Schurman, S. J. (1985). On studying emotionally hot topics: Lessons from an investigation of organizational death. In D. Berg & K. Smith (Eds.), *Clinical demands of research methods* (pp. 333-349). Beverly Hills, CA: Sage.

Van Maanen, J. (1988). *Tales of the field: On writing ethnography.* Chicago: University of Chicago Press.

Vidich, A. J., & Lyman, S. M. (1994). Qualitative methods: Their history in sociology and anthropology. In N. K. Denzin & Y. S. Lincoln (Eds.), *Handbook of qualitative research* (pp. 23-59). Thousand Oaks, CA: Sage.

Zbaracki, M. J. (1998). What people say and what people do: The rhetoric and reality of change. *Administrative Science Quarterly.*

PART 2

Processing the Researcher Experience

7

Processing the Researcher Experience Through Discussion

Susan Diemert Moch

Miriam E. Cameron

Qualitative researchers often process the researcher experience in conversation with other qualitative researchers. Such was the case with us, the authors of this chapter. Through our discussion, we decided to take the processing within ordinary conversation one step further by formally interviewing each other. This chapter describes processing the researcher experience through interviewing one another and suggests other means for processing the researcher experience.

We each had found the need to discuss our research while it was being conducted. In the situation described, we talked to each other frequently about our experiences with our research. We each had conducted phenomenological studies: Moch (1990, 1994, 1998) interviewed midlife women diagnosed with breast cancer; Cameron (1993, 1999) interviewed persons with AIDS and individuals significant to them. We were experienced interviewers and kept journals through which we examined our researcher experiences.

We often used each other as sounding boards for our research. We consulted with one another on decision making for the research. Ethical issues regarding the research became a frequent conversation topic. Sometimes, we spoke to each other about how a particular interview had been troubling or had affected us personally. Usually, when we talked, we wished for more time to explore the issues that emerged. We often discussed how we wished we had the opportunity our research respondents had—to have someone listen to each one of them in great detail and to explore the whole research experience. Therefore, we decided to schedule a significant amount of time to talk about the research and to interview each other during the scheduled time. We decided to tape-record the interviews and have them transcribed for analysis at a later time. Our real interest in conducting the interviews was to assist each other with the process of each other's respective research by sharing and reflecting on our research experiences.

Throughout the interviewing process and on further reflection about the process, we realized that the interviews served to increase understanding of the research process. More important, the interviews assisted us in gaining perspective through the difficult decision-making process with vulnerable respondents in sensitive areas of focus. For instance, Moch realized how close she was to her respondents. She felt an intimacy with them because of their talking very openly and sharing personal data. She also got very close to the respondents through the data analysis process. She realized that because of all the time she spent with the audiotapes and transcriptions, she felt she knew each respondent intimately. However, the respondents did not necessarily feel especially close to the researcher. So when she was planning to reinterview these women, whom she felt she knew very well, she wondered how it would be to be with them again. Would she somehow act closer, more intimately, than would be appropriate, given she had not interviewed them for 5 years? Cameron questioned how she should be with people who were dying and sharing intimate details of their lives with her. Several participants wanted to live on through the research, so she often felt the awesome responsibility of somehow making something of their lives. She wondered about taking from them and not giving to them in return. She spoke of her need to offer something in return to the respondents in her study. Because many of the respondents in Cameron's study were in need—physically, emotionally, and financially—it was difficult, as a researcher, not to be offering something tangible to them.

We found that sharing our research experiences through interviews was helpful. Although few publications address the benefit of participating in research interviews, many presentations include responses from participants that indicate positive experiences with interviews. We both knew the importance respondents placed on the interview process through feedback from participants in our respective research. Moch (1990) reported that participants had said they hoped Moch would do the research again in 5 years, as they liked being part of it. Other women discussed their growth and self-awareness through the interview process. The participants in Cameron's study (1997) expressed gratefulness for the opportunity to be interviewed. As one person said, "This process helped me to identify a problem and to consolidate things in my mind. To think about where I stand on the problem. I appreciate the chance to do this" (p. 30). According to a published account of the research interview (Hutchinson, Wilson, & Wilson,

1994), research participants can experience catharsis, self-acknowledgment, a sense of purpose, self-awareness, empowerment, and healing. In addition, research interviews provide a voice for persons who are disenfranchised.

Some of the benefits we found through interviewing each other included an opportunity to process the researcher experience, learning more about what participants experience through the interview, and gaining further insight for the data analysis and synthesis processes. Interviewing provided the opportunity to process the experience with someone who had gone through something similar. Sharing difficult or especially positive experiences can be helpful to the researcher who is having such a rich experience through listening to other's stories but is given no opportunity to share. The researcher often feels quite alone and isolated during the research process. Processing can provide connections with another, and this connection can be useful for data analysis. Also, insight gained through sharing the research experience can be useful in data analysis. For instance, when Moch was interviewed, she discussed past experiences with grieving in her family. She verbalized concerns that her data analysis in the breast cancer study might be overly influenced by her own experiences with grief.

Qualitative researchers who are interviewed by other skillful qualitative researchers about their research can also learn firsthand about the risks and benefits of participating in a research interview. Being a participant in the research process helps the researcher learn about feelings the respondent may possibly experience during the interview process. Sometimes, the one of us being interviewed wondered what was important to share, often taking cues from the interviewer if cues were available. Also, sometimes, the interviewee became emotional during the interview process, which increased feelings of vulnerability. When emotional responses emerged, both the interviewer and interviewee reflected on the meaning of the response for the research.

Initially, we interviewed each other about the experience of conducting the research. First, Moch interviewed Cameron about her experience of conducting the study, "Ethical Problems Experienced by Persons with AIDS." Then, Cameron interviewed Moch about her experience of conducting the study, "Living with a Diagnosis of Breast Cancer: A Five-Year Longitudinal Study." The interviews took place in Cameron's home. The interviews were audiotaped.

For each interview, the interviewer turned on the audio recorder and asked, "What is your experience of conducting this research?" Using nondirective techniques, such as, "Go on," and "Tell me more," the interviewer encouraged the interviewee to describe and examine all aspects of the question for as long as the respondent wished to talk. The interviews took 1 to 2 hours. When the interviews were finished, the interviewers talked about their experience of interviewing and listening. This conversation was also recorded and transcribed.

In addition to conducting the interviews, we analyzed the transcribed tapes after the interviews. The interviewing process and analysis methodology was derived from works by Cameron (1991), Moch (1988), Oiler (1986), Paterson and Zderad (1988), and Spiegelberg (1984).

Issues that emerged through the analysis of the interviews included the nature of the researcher-respondent relationship; ethical problems related to the research, such as the right way to structure the interviews so they would help and not harm; whether the results truly reflected the respondents; concerns about the participants' socioeconomic status and possible upcoming death; and how the experience of conducting the research impacted the meaning of life for us.

We were both pleased with our experience of participating in the interviews. Cameron described her experience of feeling understood:

> I suppose what it is, is the feeling of being understood. How much is one really understood on a deep level. That's the gift of our research. I think that they felt understood, and isn't that what we're all looking for? To feel validated that there's not something wrong with me that I have all these complicated emotions about the research participants. This is not something unique to me . . . but part of a human experience. So what you're telling me is that you hear me and that you understand what I went through and you understand on a emotional level, that's profound to me.

In addition to being intrigued and feeling energized by the experience, Moch was struck with similarities and differences in the researcher experience. As she listened to Cameron talk, she felt excited to hear what happened between Cameron and her research participants. She said, "Sometimes I thought to myself, now how is this similar or different from what I felt?"

Moch talked to Cameron about her research participants and their close calls with death. She had interviewed the same women 5 years previously, and in the course of doing the study, learned which respondents had died and which had limited prognosis at the follow-up time. Through the research and the discussion with Cameron, Moch was reminded of her own grief experiences in her life. She shared some of those with Cameron and also talked about her increased reflection about life through the research process. Moch also discussed her concern about whether she was really hearing what the respondents were saying. She shared how during the process of doing her dissertation, she became very immersed in the research and the analysis. Now, with conducting research as part of a full-time teaching position, she wondered if it was possible to immerse herself in the data to truly reflect on what the respondents were saying.

Interviewing each other was very helpful for us in processing the researcher experience. Researchers who work together on research projects may naturally discuss and process the experience through its various phases. So collaborative research may meet the need for processing the researcher experience. Other ideas for processing the researcher experience include intense conversations with another researcher. The conversations could be structured around issues related to the experience and could be scheduled so that enough time for processing would be available. Other ideas include networking with others who are doing similar research and talking in detail about the research experience.

Researchers could also write about their experience to help them deal with the research experience. We both keep journals for our research. We also keep personal journals. We have found both helpful in processing the experience. Moch found she had difficulty writing about the research experience in her research journal because of the difficulty in finding appropriate times and because of not feeling enough urgency to write about the experience. She found many things about the research experience integrated into her personal journals, however. Writing helps researchers cope with the difficult situations of the participants and also helps them experience the beauty of the participants' stories. Writing the researcher experience can also provide insight for the research findings. If, for instance, a theme keeps emerging for the researcher, the researcher must examine from where the theme emerges—the researcher's personal issues, mainly, or from both the research participant and the researcher, collaboratively.

Another possibility for processing the researcher experience is through discussion with a counselor, psychotherapist, or spiritual healer. Sometimes, participation with the respondents in the research experience makes previous emotionally laden material surface. In many situations, it is very appropriate and sometimes essential that the researcher seek support and awareness through the counseling situation.

Through this discussion on processing the researcher experience, three suggestions have been made. We interviewed each other about our respective researcher experiences with two particular studies. We found the process of being interviewed especially helpful in reflecting on the researcher experience and in making sense of the experience personally; we suggest other researchers employ this approach. Another suggestion for processing includes keeping journals about the research and incorporating feelings and thoughts about the research. In addition, researchers sometimes process the research through discussion with a counselor, psychotherapist, or spiritual healer. All processes suggested offer the researcher the opportunity to honestly deal with the reality of being affected by the research experience.

REFERENCES

Cameron, M. E. (1991). Ethical problems experienced by persons with AIDS. *Dissertation Abstracts International, 52/06B*, 2990.

Cameron, M. E. (1993). *Living with AIDS: Experiencing ethical problems.* Newbury Park, CA: Sage.

Cameron, M. E. (1997). Akrasia, AIDS, and virtue ethics. *Journal of Nursing Law, 4*(1), 21-33.

Cameron, M. E. (1999). Completing life and dying triumphantly. *Journal of Nursing Law, 6*(1), 27-32.

Hutchinson, S. A., Wilson, M. E., & Wilson, H. S. (1994). Benefits of participating in research interviews. *Image: Journal of Nursing Scholarship, 26,* 161-164.

Moch, S. D. (1988). *Health in illness: Experiences with breast cancer.* Unpublished doctoral dissertation, University of Minnesota, Minneapolis.

Moch, S. D. (1990). Health within the experience of breast cancer. *Journal of Advanced Nursing,15,* 1426-1435.

Moch, S. D. (1994, June). *Living with a diagnosis of breast cancer: A five-year longitudinal study.* Paper presented at the Qualitative Health Research Conference, Hershey, Pennsylvania.

Moch, S. D. (1998). Health-within-illness: Concept development through research and practice. *Journal of Advanced Nursing, 28*(2), 305-310.

Oiler, C. J. (1986). Phenomenology. In P. L. Munhall & C. J. Oiler (Eds.), *Nursing research: A qualitative perspective* (pp. 69-83). Norwalk, CT: Appleton-Century-Crofts.

Paterson, J. G., & Zderad, L. T. (1988). *Humanistic nursing.* New York: National League for Nursing Press.

Spiegelberg, H. (1984). *The phenomenological movement.* Boston: Martinus Nijhoff.

8

Processing Issues Related to Culture, Gender Orientation, and Mentoring

Larry E. Simmons
Marie F. Gates
Teresa L. Thompson

The focus of this chapter is on the discussion of selected processing issues that arise in relation to the experience of the researcher with the researched and with those who may be guiding the researcher who is involved with qualitative research studies for the first time. Munhall and Boyd (1993) describe the role of the qualitative researcher in terms of being a commentator on reality, enhancing the description of the presentation of reality by awareness of his or her position in the world. That position involves similarities and differences with others in that world. How these similarities and differences are recognized and reported are key to the processing of that reality.

Babbie (1983) believes that we collect and interpret qualitative data every day by the observation or participation in social behavior in academic settings, doctors' offices, waiting in airports, or anywhere. Lofland (1971) has suggested six types of social phenomena that might be assessed by a qualitative researcher: acts, activities, meanings, participation, relationships, and settings. Issues in processing qualitative information may affect all of these data collected from a variety of sources. Society assigns us formal and informal roles to play in social settings. Many of the acts, activities, meanings we assign to verbal interactions, ways we participate in settings, style of content of our interrelationships, and settings in which all of these occur are circumscribed by societal domains. In the interest of scientific explanation of a phenomenon, a qualitative researcher often must cross these arbitrary social boundaries to collect data and gather information that may describe the phenomenon of interest. Social and societal boundaries are often viewed as barriers to processing data and experiences.

In studying the other, the researcher makes choices on who he or she wishes or chooses to study. If the researcher is "unlike" the researched, the researcher may face comments such as "How could you possibly know or understand? You've not been there." There may be too many boundaries or barriers.

If the choice involves an other who is more "like" the researched, the researcher may have fewer boundaries, but the choice may lead to concerns with bias in conducting the research.

Debates regarding insider-outsider status continue when one enters the world of qualitative research. And aren't we both an insider and an outsider in any research we conduct? We believe that boundaries or barriers occur when there are differences between researcher and researched, such as gender differences or culture differences. But boundaries or barriers may also occur when the researcher and researched share so-called insider status, as may be the case with the researcher studying gender orientation. Last, boundaries may be both similar and different when mentoring occurs—particularly mentoring of graduate students hoping to learn or study qualitative methods. Mentees are researchers along with their mentors and may have much in common with them. But in their work together, the power-authority relationship affects ways that may separate them rather than unite them.

The literature and our own and others' experiences have conveyed strategies for processing the feelings, attitudes, problems, or quandaries that have been experienced in these situations. Our intent is to discuss ways to process real or artificially defined boundaries or barriers that occur when a qualitative researcher is involved in qualitative research.

DIFFERENCES BETWEEN THE RESEARCHER AND RESEARCHEE

In a recent article, Arendell (1997) presented the case for what happened when the researcher served as an interviewer in a situation where she, as a female, studied males who were undergoing divorce. She had previously studied divorced females and decided to compare the processing issues involved. Within this study, she retrospectively identified key issues related to investigating her research itself and investigating her role as researcher in the analysis. In doing so, she made the case, as feminist and critical theorists have proposed over the past decades, that "conscious subjectivity" or more open, self-reflective research has a place in conducting research, particularly of a qualitative nature. Gender in the field is a dynamic—and Arendell related examples dealing with setting the context for the interviews, such as initiating the contact and selecting the place for the interview; the men taking charge of the interview, such as jumping the gun, challenging her process of conducting the interview, being actively interviewed by the participants in the study, and overstepping boundaries in terms of checking her out; and asserting their superiority as men by such actions as denigrating women, engaging in touch behaviors, and acting in a chivalrous manner. In ending her examination, Arendell states, "Offering 'tales of the field' (Van Maanen, 1988) and subjecting our research to analytical scrutiny can move us toward greater understanding of the import of gender in group life, generally, and in research, more specifically" (p. 365).

Arendall's thought-provoking article stimulated thinking about what dynamics were operating when a bicultural, bidiscipline team engaged in a study of African Americans' lived and caring experiences with first-time diagnosis and treatment with breast cancer (Gates, Lackey, & Brown, 1996). The 13 women were recruited from clinics where the African American social work researcher practiced. The lived experiences were determined through phenomenologic interviews conducted by a Caucasian, middle-aged nurse researcher. The caring experiences were elicited through ethnographic interviews stimulated by snapshots taken by the women of caring behaviors experienced during the breast cancer experience. The second middle-aged researcher collected that data, in addition to participant-observer visits with the women in their self-selected sites that represented caring for them, such as a church service, support group, place of employment, or the clinic where they received professional service.

As a team, we came to know these women in a personal and intimate way. Their view of us at the study's end was represented by one woman's comments that "we were all in this together." The theme of commitment to women with breast cancer was a powerful one emanating from these women in terms of their need to reach out to other women in their families, at work, and at church to "do something about getting their breasts examined—and then do something about getting them treated if something bad showed up—now!" That commitment was present in the research team as well and illustrated the coparticipant relationship that the team developed with these women.

Because of that relationship, we shared feelings the women experienced in dealing with such intimate and sensitive areas as baldness, disfigurement, or sexual conflict. Feelings were similar to those described by Moch in her research with Caucasian women with breast cancer in Chapter 2. We knew several of these women would be more likely to be facing life-threatening situations due to the stage of their cancer than others. During the project, one of the women died from a separate, unrelated, and unexpected health situation. That situation shocked and devastated us. The need to support the woman's family and each other during that event was an important processing time. The fact that we were a research team provided us with the opportunity to grieve together, to recognize the importance of the woman who became so real to us, and to respond to her family and her coworkers who were also grieving her sudden death.

We marveled with the participants who reported receiving strong family and community support during the course of the study and listened attentively to the few who expressed lack of family or significant support, particularly with the men in their lives. As we analyzed and interpreted the data, we needed to recognize the importance of the feelings and insights expressed by the women in our study and their understanding of the experience. In addition, the importance of those feelings and insights directed us to learn more about whether and how the culture of the women may have contributed to the feelings and insights generated.

Literature, the clinical and cultural experience of the social work researcher, and the insights provided by our expert African American consultant knowledgeable about the culture and experienced in conducting similar research with women in another disease situation enabled us to more effectively work and process the feelings and the knowledge gained. Our consultant encouraged us to share who we were as *women* as well as *researchers* with our co-participants. For example, when one of the women asked about Gates's husband, who was in the hospital during the time of the interview, the woman offered to pray for him and said "he'll be fine." That sharing led to more extensive sharing regarding the co-participant's caring experiences during her radiation and chemotherapy treatments.

We shared our connections and our differences with our co-participants, not to burden but to let them know who we were. The quality and depth of the data reflected the quality and depth of our relationship with our co-participants.

One aspect of our study involved payment to the women. We expressed concern that the payment could subtly coerce our co-participants to become involved in the study. Our consultant helped us understand that such payment was more likely to be viewed as an indication of the worth we placed on our co-participants' time. And indeed, the co-participants spent considerable time with us. As Caucasian nurses, we were concerned that our lack of identification as African American women could hinder us in gathering the data. Again, our consultant pointed to her own research and literature supporting the view that openness, sensitivity, and development of trust were far more important considerations than identification with a specific cultural group.

Our own processing as a team involved regularly scheduled and impromptu meetings to discuss any concerns related to the conduct of the study and later, the analysis and interpretation of the findings. Because we were separately involved in the phenomenologic and ethnographic data collections, which required initial one-person analysis, then later, combined analysis with all the team members, expert advice from our second consultant, an expert in cancer research and methodology, guided us in ways to deal with the analysis that emerged and ways to incorporate the social work member who was relatively new to the research experience.

And as a team, we took time to be present for each other. If we sensed one of us had a need to vent about a troublesome situation, we did so. We planned specific times to get away from the setting itself and have fun together. One especially memorable time was high tea at the Peabody. The need for mutual support, distancing, and fun often go unstated in the processing of an intense research experience.

As we reflected on the study and thought back to Arendall's observation, our reflection led us to see that both similarities and differences played a role in the conduct and processing of the study. Arendall's openness in sharing her experiences stimulated us to wonder, for example with our study, could a man have elicited these data? We believe a man sensitive to the needs of these women, sensitive to the issues, and willing to listen could have. When funding agencies or others place restrictions on who may be the interviewer without considering the overall abilities—only looking at "sameness"—important meaning may be lost. To assume that it is the sameness of persons that determines the quality and substance of data gathered or analyzed is shortsighted. Our consultant said that what counts is the ability to listen, to hear, to be real, to know who you are so you are able to elicit the knowledge that the women are providing, and to analyze and interpret in the most open way possible.

SIMILARITY BETWEEN RESEARCHER AND RESEARCHEE: GENDER ORIENTATION

Research involving gender orientation often assumes a similarity between researcher and researched. Platzer and James (1997), in discussing methodological issues related to qualitative research involving lesbian and gay men's experiences with health care, suggested that similarity between researcher and researched is often assumed. In this section, Simmons, a doctoral candidate studying the grief experiences of HIV-negative (Simmons, 1997) and then HIV-positive (Simmons, 1999) gay men who had lost partners to AIDS, as separate cohort groups, explores several areas in relation to processing. The processing areas identified by Platzer and James (1997) include access to the community, place of interviewing, comfort with interviewing, sensitivity of questions raised, and resources used for processing.

In terms of access, the gay and lesbian communities in many metropolitan areas are recognized as cultural communities even though geographic areas do not bind them. Although often not officially recognized, these communities may have distinct social and political networks within them. Gaining access into this community may or may not present problems for the researcher who shares a similar gender orientation. When entering a community different from that of the researcher, it may prove worthwhile to ascertain if an informal structure exists that may validate the research project. Several years ago in this city, any HIV-related research needed to have the official (or unofficial, at times) backing of the leading volunteer AIDS service organization in the city. But that organization does not hold the credibility or value that it once had within the gay community, and sponsorship of that particular agency is no longer a prerequisite for entry into the community. Another organization has emerged as the predominant agency in AIDS care, but the gay community does not value this political agency as it once did the all-volunteer agency in the early years of the AIDS crisis.

In both of the studies identified, access to the client population went smoothly. With the first study, involving the HIV-negative group (Simmons, 1997), the process went slowly and took more time. Concern was expressed that although it may have been easy to get access to HIV-negative men, it might not be so easy to find HIV-positive men who would be willing to talk about the situation. Four sites providing health care and social services for HIV-infected persons were involved. I had established personal connections with workers in those sites. When the recruitment began for the second study (Simmons, 1999), I was flooded with calls from potential participants for the study. Believing that I needed to interview these men as quickly as possible to obtain all the participants, I collected the data in 6 weeks. My ability to process and be real to these men was greatly affected by the pace of doing the interviews. "Easy" access proved to a barrier for me in not allowing the time to process the data, reflect, and relate at the level needed as a researcher.

The interview setting itself presented another issue. An "insider" in the gay community, for example, may choose an interview setting or ask the participant to choose an interview setting that is more comfortable for the participant, such as a coffee house, gay bar, or in the home of a gay couple. But the comfort level of the interviewer during the data collection where the setting is more public or noisy may become an issue. For example, a participant in my HIV-positive group who had lost his partner to AIDS 1 month earlier (Simmons, 1999) requested that the interview take place in a local chain restaurant rather than at his home. The interview was held at the restaurant but proved to be distracting for me as the interviewer, with servers coming and going by the table, people talking, customers entering and leaving. The audiotape of the interview was also difficult for the transcriber to understand. Now that I have had that experience, I believe that the participant's choice of setting for the interview is still primary, but suggesting a less busy time for the meeting would permit accommodation for both interviewer and interviewee needs.

Establishing rapport and gaining trust, of course, were extremely important. Planning interviews in the home setting more readily promoted that type of ambience. Having worked in home nursing care areas for many years, my comfort level in going into homes was fairly high, although I always remained very respectful of the wishes of the person that I was visiting. In data collection for my first study, interviews with grieving HIV-negative men (Simmons, 1997), the comfort level may have been a positive factor in the amount and type of information relayed to me during the interviews. When typing the transcript for one of my interviews, for example, the transcriptionist was often amazed at how much information was given. With the opening question, one participant talked for what transcribed to be 12 pages. The transcriptionist remarked, "I don't think that he even took a breath!" Whether it was my comfort level at being there and asking a question that nobody else had ever asked or my listening skills and abilities that enabled me to collect so much data, or a combination of both, I believe that the comfortable setting contributed to the data obtained.

In contrast to the first study, in my second study involving the grief experienced by HIV-positive gay partners of men who died (Simmons, 1999), I found I was not so comfortable. This discomfort was exacerbated by my decision to interview all who responded to the request, without sufficient time to breathe. The ease in obtaining access led to an urgency in data collection, which ultimately affected my ability to process what was happening to me as I interviewed so many of these men so quickly.

As I interviewed, I was overly conscious of overt reactions on my part to what was being said or observed. Knowing that these men could be sensitive to what may be perceived as negative reactions to them or what they said led me to purposefully not react when participants in this study would describe, for example, unsafe sexual behaviors in which they engaged after the death of the partner. I assumed a negative reaction, either by physical response or verbal response, may have interfered with the rest of the interview. I would go back to the issue for clarification purposes but tried very hard not to attach any message to my questioning that would be taken as disapproval or of judging their actions. As a result, I did not take into account how my reactions were affecting me as I heard so many stories and so much pain expressed in so short a time. My usually excellent interviewing skills were not being used as carefully as in the past. I did not pursue feelings or experiences, as I found I did in the first study.

I reflected back on who I turned to for support during the first phase of the study. I turned to friends, family, peers, and established qualitative researchers to help work through issues that concerned me. Had a consultant been used on the project, ongoing discussion with that consultant would have been helpful. When I have assisted others with data analysis, they have also used me as a sounding board or listener on their studies. The connection with someone else who understands the data and methodology appeared to have been quite invaluable to them. When I presented the preliminary data from my first gay male grief study (Simmons, 1997), the questions and feedback I received at the conference were most valuable to me in analyzing the data and findings for accuracy.

However, as I reflect on the second study, whose findings are currently undergoing analysis (Simmons, 1999), it would have been helpful for me to consider securing a specific processing person or counselor. The person could have helped me to identify issues that were troublesome for me in data collection (e.g., talking about safer sex or discussing what was happening to me as I inundated myself with so many interviews so quickly). As I look back on my interviews, I can see areas I was afraid to address—afraid for myself and afraid of leaving the men with issues and no support person.

MENTORING ISSUES

Simmons's experience leads into a discussion regarding what happens when doctoral students who often have been skilled clinicians become involved with a study that deals with sensitive issues and may or may not involve dealing with a population of which they feel a part. Thompson and Gates recalled an opportunity they had with a cohort of doctoral student colleagues to process experiences with an experienced mentor, skilled not only in qualitative methods but in dealing with issues related to those methods that needed addressing. Doctoral study presents an opportunity for students engaged in study with an established mentor to have the opportunity to process theoretical, design, and interpersonal issues involved in conducting qualitative research. Gates and Thompson (1993) presented a paper at the Midwest Nursing Research Society in which they shared strategies used as doctoral students to process, with an experienced research mentor, what has been happening as they conducted their individual studies. Informal sessions between the mentor and the six students enabled the group, who had chosen to use ethnographic, ethnonursing designs in conducting their studies, the opportunity to learn together. This opportunity provided the students with the time and space to explore the framework, decide on design, work out the specific data collection methods, prepare ways to analyze their data, and so forth. The students were instrumental in helping to develop the Leininger-Templin-Thompson (1992) data software that assisted their mentor and themselves in coding the data. This experience enabled students to challenge ideas, suggest different approaches, and understand how to develop and use a qualitative design. Students could bring back their concerns in terms of generating problems; trying out interview formats; role-playing with one another in designing and conducting interviews; critiquing each other's data; gaining skill and experience in coding, analyzing, and interpreting data; and helping each other with writing.

At the time, the students were not aware of how much support they provided to each other in listening to the struggles involved in dealing with identification of caring behaviors with persons from other cultures, such as old-order Amish (Wenger, 1988); Lebanese Muslim immigrants (Luna, 1993); Philippine American nurses (Spangler, 1992); or with tackling sensitive issues related to caring, such as Anglo-Canadian nurses caring for disabled husbands (Cameron, 1990) or patients who were dying in hospital and hospice settings (Gates, 1991); or understanding the trials and tribulations of newly admitted and long-term residents in rehabilitation settings (Thompson, 1990). Their ability to understand and assist each other even enabled one of the students to pinch-hit for another at an Institutional Review Board hearing, when a sudden life-threatening emergency occurred. Familiarity with the study and with each other provided that advantage.

Along with theoretical and research issues, they could help each other see when they needed breaks, when time off was necessary, when they needed outside support, when they might be getting too close to their data, or when their own personal experiences might be affecting what was happening in their studies. As one example, Gates's 11-year-old nephew was diagnosed and subsequently died of cancer shortly after she defended the proposal for her study. Personal events certainly affected what was going on, and the support of the doctoral team and faculty mentor provided her with helpful guidance and support to get through it, including her decision to take some time away from the situation and leave the dissertation alone for awhile to spend time with her brother and his family.

An important part of the support given to each other included ways to strengthen the defense of their ideas for including specific data important to the dissertation or maintaining the integrity of using specific metaphors to characterize the analysis, rather than backing down when working with their faculty mentors. The team members' experiences in processing stimulated each of them to continue supporting others who were conducting qualitative studies, whether in clinical or academic settings.

Reflection on our mentoring experiences suggests that doctoral students need opportunities to be able to speak with each other as a necessary part of getting through the experience with a doctoral committee. This is not intended in any way to disparage mentors who are guiding students in the difficult areas of qualitative research. Mentors are essential and critical. But there may be times when students require the time and space to explore concerns, particularly those of a personal nature, with like-minded persons or peer groups. It may be necessary, then, for the student to find someone knowledgeable with the process, but not in a power position, to help ease and enrich the dissertation process. Power distribution in the mentor-student relationship may preclude the student from raising in that context all the issues he or she may wish to address. It is helpful to have colleagues with whom to debrief when sensitive issues arise.

CONCLUSION

We have discussed selected issues related to gender, culture, and mentoring in the processing of qualitative research. Boundaries, whether real or artificial, should not discourage the qualitative researcher. Identification of issues or potential issues and increased awareness of issues when performing all phases of the process are necessary and take time. Developing a plan to confront, alleviate, and process issues during all phases of qualitative research requires time, energy, and thought.

REFERENCES

Arendell, T. (1997). Reflections on the researcher-researched relationship: A woman interviewing men. *Qualitative Sociology, 20*, 341-368.

Babbie, E. (1983). *The practice of social research* (3rd ed.). Belmont, CA: Wadsworth.

Cameron, C. F. (1990). *An ethnonursing study of the influence of extended caregiving on the health status of elderly Anglo-Canadian widows caring for disabled husbands.* Unpublished dissertation, Wayne State University, Detroit, Michigan.

Gates, M. F. (1991). Transcultural comparison of hospital and hospice as caring environments for dying patients. *Journal of Transcultural Nursing, 2*(2), 3-15.

Gates, M. F., Lackey, N. R., & Brown, G. (1996). *Black women's lived/caring experiences with breast cancer: Final report.* Memphis, TN: Oncology Nursing Foundation.

Gates, M. F., & Thompson, T. C. L. (1993, March 27). *Guiding ourselves and others in ways of knowing and doing qualitative research.* Poster presentation given to the Midwest Nursing Research Society, Cleveland, Ohio.

Leininger, M. M., Templin, T., & Thompson, F. (1992). *The Leininger-Templin-Thompson ethnoscript qualitative software program.* Detroit, MI: Wayne State University.

Lofland, J. (1971). *Analyzing social settings.* Belmont, CA: Wadsworth.

Luna, L. (1993). Care and cultural context of Lebanese Muslim immigrants using Leininger's theory. *Journal of Transcultural Nursing, 5*(2), 12-20.

Munhall, P. L., & Boyd, C. O. (1993). *Nursing research: A qualitative perspective.* New York: National League for Nursing Press.

Platzer, H., & James, T. (1997). Methodological issues conducting sensitive research on lesbian and gay men's experience of nursing care. *Journal of Advanced Nursing, 25*, 626-633.

Simmons, L. E. (1997, March). *The lived grief experience of HIV-negative gay men who lost a partner to AIDS.* Paper presented at Midwest Nursing Research Society, Minneapolis, Minnesota.

Simmons, L. E. (1999). *The grief experience of HIV-positive gay men who lose partners to AIDS.* Unpublished doctoral dissertation, University of Missouri at Kansas City.

Spangler, Z. (1992). Transcultural care values and nursing practices of Philippine-American nurses. *Journal of Transcultural Nursing, 3*(2), 28-37.

Thompson, T. L. C. (1990). *A qualitative investigation of rehabilitation nursing care in an inpatient rehabilitation unit using Leininger's theory.* Unpublished dissertation, Wayne State University, Detroit, Michigan.

Van Maanen, J. (1988). *Tales of the field: On writing ethnography.* Chicago: University of Chicago Press.

Wenger, A. F. Z. (1988). *The phenomenon of care in a high context culture: The old order Amish.* Unpublished dissertation, Wayne State University, Detroit, Michigan.

9

Qualitative Researchers Working as Teams

Marie F. Gates
Pamela S. Hinds

Research teams involve more than one person working on a study. Qualitative research teams are defined by some researchers as the dyad of the researcher and the participant or informant. However, our meaning of *team* in this chapter is when more than a single person is in the role of the researcher while studying the same topic in a collaborative or joint manner. Such teams are becoming more common because of the expanded scope of studies, a recognized need for diverse viewpoints when crafting a study and analyzing data, and because more hands (and more heads) are needed to do the work of a study. Although there is a growing body of literature that addresses benefits, challenges, and issues related to selecting and developing research teams (Adler & Adler, 1987; Grady & Wallston, 1988), only a few reports address these for research teams engaged in a qualitative study (Allen & Walker, 1992; Erickson & Stull, 1998; Pickett, Brennan, Greenberg, Licht, & Worrell, 1994, Tripp-Reimer, Sorofman, Peters, & Waterman, 1994).

This chapter explores selected situations involving qualitative research teams and will offer general strategies to benefit the team and the research. These strategies relate to selecting study sites and team members, selecting the construct or process to be studied, and for selecting the research method. More specifically, this chapter highlights strategies for (a) developing and maintaining a team at one site, which consists of members from the same discipline; (b) expanding an established team to include a member from another discipline; and (c) establishing studies involving multisite, multidisciplinary teams. Challenges and opportunities experienced by teams conducting qualitative research are presented through examples of the work from different teams.

SAME-DISCIPLINE TEAMS
AT THE SAME SITE

This section describes the formation of a same-discipline team at one site as it evolved into a partnership. Development of the team through processing strategies related to supporting each other during the conduct of the research is discussed first, followed by processing strategies related to supporting other professional and personal commitments.

Developing the Research Team
and Interest Area

Lackey and Gates, two nurse researchers, began their tenure at the same university more than 7 years ago. Their entry into the system at the same time, and the support of the university for joint research endeavors, stimulated their initial idea of collaboration. Similarities of research interests—namely, care of adult patients with cancer in clinic, home, and hospice settings—and expertise in qualitative methods further facilitated their eventual decision to form a research team. The team's first study (Lackey & Gates, 1994) focused on a comparative description of needs of patients with cancer, their caregivers, and their families. The study was conducted in clinics and hospice settings in a large Southern city and its environs.

While working on this first study (Lackey & Gates, 1994), the researchers gained familiarity with settings, resources, and people. More important, both identified a number of youngsters who were involved with the caregiving of adult patients with cancer. That observation, along with Lackey's earlier awareness of youngsters giving care to adults in a different population and Gates' identification of that same phenomenon in her community health nursing experiences, led to their decision to focus on young caregivers (ages 8-18) caring for adult patients with cancer at home. As the team grappled with the phenomenon and became aware of the limited research in the area, they decided that study of the young caregiver was a necessary and fruitful area for research. They were delighted to discover that each had experience in different qualitative approaches, which allowed them to study this relatively unexplored phenomenon more fully: Lackey with phenomenology and Gates with ethnography. These two complementary approaches would enable them to gain some breadth and depth of knowledge about the questions proposed for the study: (a) What was the experience of caregiving like for these youngsters and (b) what effects did the caregiving have on the youngsters' life ways, family life, school, and other activities? Because the team had been recently involved with the patient needs study, they decided to add the unstructured survey to the other qualitative approaches to add the dimension of needs identified by these young caregivers (Gates & Lackey, 1998; Lackey & Gates, 1997).

Team Development During
Conduct of the Study

Team development was fostered by the data collection experience. The team decided that both researchers would meet with the families together, to describe the sequential nature of the data collection, including the need for family consent as well as youngster assent. At the end of this visit, Lackey arranged the time for the first interview, to be conducted by Lackey alone, which focused on enabling the youngster to talk about his or her feelings and experiences related to caring for the parent or grandparent with cancer. At the end of her talking with the youngster, Lackey asked the child to list his or her needs as a young caregiver of an adult with cancer. Gates then arranged her visit(s) to conduct the ethnographic interviews and participant observation. Times to observe and participate with the youngster in caregiving and other events, such as school, church, and extracurricular activities, were included. The team engaged in constant contact as an essential feature of this investigation, keeping detailed notes regarding communication, design, data collection, and data management.

The team also made the decision to analyze each data set separately and to combine the analyses later. In combining the analyses, richer, fuller description of the phenomenon was obtained. For example, the youngsters provided the researcher with a phenomenological description of caregiving with its emotional overlay, whereas the ethnographic data yielded the categorization of the caregiving task and varying roles of caregiving assumed within the milieu of the family. The depth and scope of the types of caregiving could be confirmed by both the phenomenologic and ethnographic analyses. Divergences also became apparent as the data were analyzed together. For example, each of the youngsters in multiple-caregiver families claimed to "do the most" in the phenomenologic data set, contrasted with the older child having the greater responsibility, as elicited from the ethnographic interviews and observations. The painstaking work of the combined analyses led to identifying specific areas requiring further exploration, such as decision-making rules, authority, and the process by which youngsters becoming engaged in caregiving tasks. (For a fuller description, including representation of the matrix depicting the contributions made by the separate and combined analyses, see Lackey & Gates, 1997).

The regularly scheduled time spent in planning the study, conducting the study, and in combining the separately analyzed data sets fostered the development of this same-discipline team. The team viewed the scheduled team meeting times as absolute commitments—similar to classes, committee meetings, or other regularly scheduled appointments. The sacrosanct time provided the team with structure for the work of the team and opportunity to learn about work habits, styles, and perspectives. The team found commonalities related to the conduct of research and the way work is done—each was willing to "do her share," to work on weekends or in the evening if the need arose, to be true to the methods chosen, and to conduct the research with integrity. Listening respectfully to one another's ideas, even if disagreeing about a way to handle things, was an important commonality. Respectful listening could lead to a change in research operation. For example, Lackey was amused by Gates's ethnographic strategy of writing up field notes. Through ongoing discussion about the value of the field notes, Lackey eventually consented to keeping a journal detailing additional observations and comments and her feelings and responses to the data, and she conceded that this strategy did indeed add to her completeness in recording and in analyzing the phenomenological data. Two excellent consultants, in qualitative methodology and child-adolescent development aided the processing through insightful questions aimed at shaping and extending the work being done.

The team has found its greatest struggle to be in writing up the study results and developing manuscripts. Rather than working separately on writing, the team has found it useful to use planned times together for writing, either working together on a particularly knotty section of a manuscript or separately on separate sections of an article or proposal. The opportunity to say "what do you think about this piece—I'm not getting it quite right" has been helpful in developing the writing pieces. The planned times kept each person motivated to get on with that work.

Following the completion of that study and during the development of manuscripts, the team worked on a more extensive proposal related to youngster caregiving. While working on that proposal, the team completed another study detailing the retrospective experiences of adults who had been child caregivers of their parents or grandparents with a variety of chronic physical illnesses, including cancer. Insights provided by adults who had engaged in caregiving as children are expected to add greater understanding to potential depth that may be added to other studies dealing with child caregivers within the family context.

Additional Processes Related to Team Development

In addition to work times, our team found it helpful to build in celebration times—for example, for receipt of a teaching award or a birthday—to foster greater awareness of who we are in roles different from researcher. Through personal crises each of us has experienced—deaths of close family members, family illnesses, stresses occurring in other aspects of our work lives—the team has become sensitive to each other's need for a listening ear, an offer to sit with an ill family member, a sudden trip to the airport, all of which have solidified the growing respect, trust, and "counting on each other," which have evolved in the partnership. Times spent with each other away from the research have helped the team identify differences in personality or background that could affect how interactions occur. For example, Lackey was raised in a small, rural farming community with other family members close by but not too close. Gates, on the other hand, grew up in a 5-room upper flat in Hamtramck, a Polish American community surrounded by Detroit. That kind of awareness helped each to understand one's greater need for space and solitary time and the other's comfort amid clutter, closeness, and lots of people. Including times for play, relaxation, and times to get to know each other assists in processing between team members. Erickson and Stull (1998) identify lessons important for teams to learn as they work together: trust, responsibility, and complementarity. The processes used in the conduct of the research itself and in other interactions helped this team to learn and use those lessons.

EXPANDING A SAME-DISCIPLINE PARTNERSHIP TO AN INTERDISCIPLINARY TEAM: SAME SITE

As lessons learned helped us identify the positive nature of research teams, those lessons stimulated openness in including others in the team configuration. In conducting the two earlier studies, the team became acquainted with Brown, a social worker at one of the clinics. Brown was instrumental in facilitating early entry into the clinic for the patient-caregiver-family needs study (Lackey & Gates, 1994) and in suggesting names of several families with young caregivers for the second study (Gates & Lackey, 1998).

Developing the Expanded Research Team and Interest Area

Brown's professional manner, her interest and concern for patients and families, her skill in developing support groups for women with breast cancer, and her exciting work in fostering programs to promote African American women's decisions to seek screening and treatment for breast cancer encouraged early interactions of the team with Brown. Several conversations with her led to the consideration of developing a joint project. Because all of us had strong concerns for African American women with breast cancer and ways to promote early diagnosis and treatment, an opportunity presented itself to consider formation of a broader team. The two-member team suggested to Brown the possibility of becoming a three-member team. The joint partnership had complementary professional interests and broadened the scope of the team by adding the disciplinary approach of social work, the African American cultural perspective, and a more clinical focus to approaching this area of study.

A descriptive, exploratory study was eventually proposed to (a) examine the day-to-day life of African American women with breast cancer, (b) determine the caring behaviors given and received by the women during this experience, and (c) to explore possible relationships between caring and delay in seeking and continuing treatment for cancer. The caring aspect was a jointly agreed-on speculation regarding African American women's delay in seeking treatment.

Team Development During Conduct of the Study

The exploratory nature of the study suggested the use of qualitative approaches to identify the experience of women newly diagnosed with breast cancer (phenomenology) and to explore how caring for and from others may or may not contribute to seeking and maintaining treatment (ethnography). Brown was eager to contribute. Although not trained in research methods beyond her graduate work, Brown was eager to learn and saw her role prominently in identifying women for the study, explaining the study, and exploring alternative sites for recruitment. She initially expressed reluctance regarding involvement with the analysis and interpretation phases, but encouragement to do so eased her concerns.

Brown approached participants on visits to the clinic, explained the study in detail, and obtained agreement for participation. Lackey made the first contact in the participants' homes for the phenomenologic visit. Following those interviews, she and Gates made a joint visit to explain that a camera would be used to take snapshots and subsequent ethnographic interviews would relate to the snapshots and participant-observation opportunities. When the snapshots were taken, a copy was given to each participant for purposes of eliciting meaning, kinds and extent of generic caring given and received by the participant. Arrangements were made for the participant-observation visit, with the women selecting either a work setting, health care setting, religious group, or support group. Again, to be true to the methods of phenomenology and ethnography, the team agreed it was important and necessary for the members who knew those methods to collect the data and analyze the specific data sets. Included in the ethnographic data were recorded notes of team conferences and visits with methodology and culture consultants.

Analysis of the data led to a phenomenologic description of their lived experience by African American women and ethnographic identification of caring themes related to caring for and from others, along with potential themes related to delay: care provider "wait and see" watchfulness, horror stories related to side effects or treatment, and reticence or resignation related to trusting in the Lord and not talking about seeking treatment, particularly in the older women. Combining data again led to confirmation of findings between data sets, with a special openness brought about by the women's involvement with the snapshot taking. One of the strongest findings was the belief by the women in the study that, as one woman said in referring to the researchers and participants, "all of us were in this together." That declaration was one of affirmation of the team of researchers with the team of participants as one large team.

Regularly scheduled meetings among the three members were critical to the smooth conduct of the study. Consistency in recruiting and in the approach to the women in following the protocol was necessary because participants were likely to see each other at other times: for example, during chemotherapy sessions. Same-site conferences with the consultant who was in town fostered the discussion of the team in conducting the study and in preparing for the separate and joint analyses. Telephone conferences with the team's consultant on African American issues affirmed strategies for promoting cohesiveness in research and participant team development, for recognizing the value of offering stipends for participation in the study, and for affirming the qualities of openness, trust development, and respect as important in conducting the study. Brown's clinical insights and alliances with the community contributed helpful insight into the analysis and interpretations of the findings. Her expressed comfort with the team and with both consultants contributed to her role in that regard.

Additional Processes Related to Team Development

As we did before, building in social times for lunch or dinner together to explore not only working relationships but also who we were in our individual lives helped to maintain working relationships. Brown's interest in raising African violets coincided with Lackey's gardening skills. Both tended to tease Gates about her "brown thumb." Brown and Gates tended to share experiences related to their young adult children. Professional processes also aided the team's growth. Brown would call on the nurses of the team for advice or resources related to her clients or herself. In addition to her research, Brown played a pivotal role in assisting the researchers in working with graduate students interested in conducting studies in Brown's clinic site. In addition to their research efforts, Gates and Lackey assisted Brown in her support and prevention groups through volunteer activities with both groups. These efforts were examples of our support for each other's additional professional activities.

At this writing, the final report of the study (Gates, Lackey, & Brown, 1996) has been filed. Manuscripts have been sent for review. That process has been delayed by two members' move from the geographic site and the third member's move from her specific clinic site. However, the team has reaffirmed its commitment to each work more diligently to see that the stories of the participants in this study are told. In addition, Brown has asked for assistance in preparing a clinical article related to her development of breast cancer support groups. Times to accomplish both of those assignments have been set.

The combining of the two disciplines of social work and nursing has led to opportunities to share complementarity in the team's commitment to the women in this study, genuine concern for them in hearing their stories, the team's viewing of them as co-participants in the research enterprise, and a dedication to complete the ongoing work so that their stories will be told.

Each of these instances—development of a same-discipline team at the same site and expanding the partnership to include another discipline at the same site—present a serendipitous coming together of people who then decided to become teams and worked together in developing and maintaining those teams. In both situations, the conscious working together of the people involved contributed to the strengthening of the teams, such that even though the members are no longer in the same place, they continue to maintain their relationships. The next section describes the establishing of teams at different sites and explores a conscious decision to develop a multisite team for conducting qualitative research.

ESTABLISHING TEAMS TO CONDUCT MULTISITE QUALITATIVE RESEARCH STUDIES

There are three components that need to be addressed prior to initiating a multisite qualitative research study, each of which involves a careful selection process. The selections include team and site members, construct or process, and qualitative research method. Once these selections are completed, concentrated attention must be given to developing a committed, interactive team that will maximize the descriptive and explanatory meaning of the study data. A successful qualitative multisite research team is able to accurately and sensitively detect the studied construct or process and identify differences and similarities in its context across geographically distinct settings. Such differences and similarities contribute to our understanding of the studied construct or process and are a special benefit of conducting multisite qualitative studies. Brief descriptions of the three selection processes follow. Then, two examples of multisite qualitative studies are included to illustrate the three selection processes.

Selecting Team Members and Sites

The selection process of team members involves identifying individual researchers who have expertise in the use of qualitative research methodologies and who enjoy a group approach to research using such methods. This enjoyment means being comfortable in sharing and discussing analytical impressions, surmisings, and hypotheses. This careful selection of team members includes a purposeful seeking of diversity in perspectives and perhaps in life experiences. The combination of expertise with methodology, interest in the construct or process, comfort with the group approach, and diversity of perspectives and life experiences will foster the analytical approach desired to learn the essential attributes and multiple facets of the construct or process under study. This triangulation of researchers (or multiple observers with different experiences who are occupying equally prominent roles in the analytical process) enhances the opportunity to identify more about the construct or process under study than a lone researcher at a single site. A unique benefit of creating a team of diverse members is that the conceptual biases of a single team member are likely to be compensated for by different biases in another team member (Denzin, 1989; Lincoln & Guba, 1985). It is also quite likely that in the analytical process, the biases of each team member will be identified, and discussions about those will contribute to the development of each individual team member as a qualitative researcher.

Characteristics of settings also need to be considered when selecting team members. Final selections are made from a matrix of setting and researcher characteristics. Characteristics of settings that merit consideration include their administrators' respect for qualitative research methodologies, serious interest in the construct or process that will be the focus of the research, ability to commit resources (especially researcher's time) to a multisite study, and willingness to seriously reflect on differences and similarities in the study findings that are site specific.

Selecting the Construct or Process

The next selection process includes selecting the construct or process that will be studied by the team. Constructs of a private or deeply personal nature, such as studying the researcher's response to abuse or violence or experience with a perceived failure, may not lend themselves to a multisite team approach. The danger with these types of constructs is that they may evoke strong personal interpretations and not theoretical analyses. Team members may vacillate between assuming therapeutic roles with each other and research roles with the data. The basic conflict here is that a therapist attempts to develop an individual, including his or her strengths and realistic self-perceptions, whereas a researcher attempts to develop ideas, and indirectly, people. Role confusion about being the therapist or the researcher will confound interpreting data and confuse the process of data generation with actual findings.

Selecting the Research Method

The third selection process is directed at the qualitative research method. Although the selection of method is primarily dictated by the research question itself, it is influenced by the qualities, talents, and expertise of the team members, as well as by the characteristics of the study settings. For example, the phrasing of the research question will reflect what is already known about the construct, the purpose of the proposed research, the collective research expertise of the team members, and the setting administration's understanding or appreciation of the method. Nuances of a construct or process are more likely to be captured if the researchers are expert in the selected method. However, some administrations are not as tolerant of iterative research processes as others and insist on exact sampling techniques and methodological detail being specified in advance. For example, a scientific review board at a particular setting may require that all of the interview questions be specified in advance of approving the study. Such a requirement will necessarily direct a research team away from a grounded theory methodology to a semistructured interview format. Thus, a compromise of method and purpose may be forged in such a situation.

Example #1: Grounded Theory Study of
Coping With a Return of a Child's Cancer

The purpose of this three-site study was to identify the process that parents and their children who were receiving treatment for cancer experienced when the child's cancer returned after it was thought to be cured. Three researchers with strong experience using grounded theory methodology and who had additional expertise in family development, family adaptation to chronic illness, and child and adolescent responses to health threats were chosen to lead research teams at their respective sites. Personal traits of these three researchers that further promoted their selection included perseverance and high energy levels.

Also considered in the matrix of researcher and setting characteristics for this study was the previous positive support in the respective settings for qualitative research methodologies, an expressed strong interest in parents' and patients' coping with recurrence of disease, and expressed interest in developing a multi-disciplinary team to conduct a study on this topic. We chose to exclude settings that rarely treat recurrent cancer and to include families who were being treated for the second time at the same treatment setting so that unfamiliar setting and staff would not be a factor influencing the evolving theory.

The three teams determined that the team led by the researcher with the most extensive experience with the research method would conduct the first interview and then distribute the transcription to the other two site coordinators. The site coordinators took advantage of a national meeting that they were all attending to jointly review the transcribed interview, share impressions of the data from their unique perspectives, initiate first-level coding, and comment on the interviewing style of the researcher. This format of sharing the transcripts and first-level coding continued with every interview that was completed at each of the three sites.

Interactions of an analytical nature were facilitated by each site using the same computer software to manage interview data. In addition, conference calls were held every 6 to 8 weeks to review evolving impressions as a result of conducting the interviews and analyzing the transcribed interview data and field notes from all three sites. These frequent conference calls had benefit beyond analyzing the meaning of the data. They were a definite source of support for the individual team efforts at the respective sites and helped the site-based teams become more cohesive as individual groups and more committed to the study. Individual frustrations were shared during these calls and were met with team suggestions and support. Dilemmas about staff concerns or patient and family responses to the questions were also dealt with on a regular basis.

An agenda was forwarded to each team leader in advance of each conference call, and a set of minutes regarding the discussions and decisions was forwarded to each site following the conference call. Towards the end of the first year of data collection, an unusual situation arose at one site. The team leader indicated that she would have limited time to dedicate to the study for several months. She anticipated being able to enroll and interview patients but not to analyze the resulting data. The agreement achieved during a conference call of the team leaders was that the transcribed interviews would be forwarded to the principal investigator of the study who would assume responsibility for coding the interviews. The coded interviews were discussed during the regularly scheduled conference calls and then returned to the team leader who had conducted the interview for her final review and additional input. This continued for six interviews. Had this happened at an earlier point in the team-building process, this arrangement might not have been feasible. Only because the team leaders had worked closely together could another member assist temporarily in this way.

An agenda item included in each conference call was feedback on interviewing skills. After each interview was analyzed in terms of its content meaning, each was reviewed for flow of content and influence of interviewer style on interviewee responses. Each team leader agreed that this particular agenda item assisted in refining her interview skills. Other standing agenda items were (a) the functioning of respective teams at each site, (b) study participants' reactions to the study, and (c) the impact of conducting the interviews and overseeing the study on the team leaders. It was also during these telephone conference calls that probes for further refinement of emerging codes and categories were discussed and agreed on. The success of the previously developed probes was discussed. The frequency and the intensity of these telephone discussions contributed to the timely saturation of the emerging categories and substantive-level theory.

A unique benefit for the team leaders in conducting the multisite grounded theory study involved self-examination of individual styles when approaching patients and their parents about enrolling in the study. One particular site had a higher refusal rate than the other two sites. Careful discussions among the team leaders about the difference included consideration of environmental and researcher characteristics that could influence the refusal rate. Discussions focused on the tentativeness of the team leader when discussing the topic of recurrence with families who seemed likely to refuse to participate in the study. Joint review of the first few interviews completed at the other two sites assisted the team leader in identifying the positive outcomes of participating in the study for patients and parents. During a period of low study enrollment at this site, the team leader remarked that she continued to feel a part of the study and the larger team because she was able to code the interviews being conducted at the other two sites. This sharing helped the team member remain committed to the study and to become more comfortable with the construct being studied.

All sites concurrently initiated validation interviews. This was a time of special excitement for the team leaders and members as field notes and interview responses were discussed during conference calls. The same process of regularly scheduled conference calls was used to develop the manuscripts that reported study findings (Birenbaum, Hinds, & Clarke-Steffen, 1995; Hinds et al., 1996).

Example #2: Using Focus Groups to Study
Three Perspectives on Fatigue in Children

The purpose of this two-site study was to identify the essential characteristics of fatigue in 7- to 12-year-old children who were receiving treatment for cancer. Three perspectives (patient, parent, and health care professionals) on the fatigue were solicited because fatigue is theorized to be a symptom whose management is directly influenced by the beliefs and knowledge of others surrounding the child. A qualitative approach was chosen because a conceptual definition of fatigue did not exist for this specific patient group. Lacking that, accurate clinical assessments of fatigue in these children could not be conducted. As a result, a potentially treatable symptom that was reported by patients as causing difficulties in their ability to function (play, concentrate at school, have adequate nutritional intake, take part in conversations) was not being addressed (Hinds et al., 1999; Hockenberry-Eaton et al., 1998).

The two sites were selected because of the strong leadership of a nurse researcher in each site who had established research programs involving symptom management and because of the size of the pediatric oncology program at each site that permitted ready access to a large sample of patients in the target age group. Team members from the two sites were purposely selected to reflect the overall project intention of establishing a clinical scholars program. The scholars, who were already expert in the care of the child with cancer, would learn the additional skills of conducting and translating research on symptom management into direct patient care. The teams at both sites were led by nurse researchers who had experience with qualitative methodologies, including the use of focus groups. The intentional combination of clinical and research experts on the study teams also reflected the anticipated need to solicit clinical accounts on fatigue from health care professionals who might be unaware of their clinical knowledge on this symptom. Fellow clinicians, carefully trained to conduct focus group interviews, were expected to be particularly effective in soliciting participation from other health care staff, pediatric oncology patients, and parents. The ultimate aims of this program were to (a) clarify misperceptions about fatigue that are held by patients, parents, and staff; (b) assist health care professionals, parents, and patients in detecting and assessing the fatigue, and to (c) implement effective interventions. The nature of these aims seemed most legitimately addressed by the combined talents of the researchers and clinicians.

The research method selected was that of semistructured interviews with established prompts. Transcripts of the focus groups were analyzed using content analytical techniques (Krippendorff, 1980). This approach was purposely chosen because more descriptive information about fatigue from the three perspectives (parent, patient, and health care professional) is needed and because a more structured method for data collection would lend itself to use by clinical scholars across the two sites. Workshops for the team members on conducting focus groups were held at the beginning of the study and were followed by periodic review of the methodology in team meetings. Participants at each site assumed three different roles (facilitator, observer, participant) during those workshops and follow-up sessions. In addition, a teleconference session between the two sites was held regarding the methodology.

Interactions of an analytical nature were facilitated by additional teleconferences, joint meetings at national meetings, telephone exchanges, and almost daily E-mail messages between the two nurse researchers. An ambitious plan for conducting the research and distributing study findings was agreed to by both teams and is credited by the teams with keeping them focused on each milestone within the plan. The blend of talents from the teams also contributed to the analysis of data. One team had more conceptual leanings, and the other, more clinical leanings. When merged, these two potential biases assisted the research teams in extracting additional meaning from the abstract nuances and implications, as well as the concrete detail in the evolving data set.

The transcripts from the first two focus groups were jointly coded by the two nurse researchers. They then created a coding dictionary, and at least two team members from each site coded the subsequently transcribed focus group interviews. The three perspectives (patient, parent, health care professionals) were solicited at both sites through the focus groups, but after the initial coding dictionary was developed, each site was assigned chief responsibility for the coding and interpretation of the data for a certain perspective (i.e., site 1 was responsible for the patient and parent data; site 2 was responsible for the health care professional data). This division of responsibilities was purposeful so that the respective teams could concentrate on one perspective and have a greater ability to detect differences by site within that perspective. The division of responsibilities also assisted in distributing the burdens secondary to coding the data and increased the team's familiarity with the assigned data set. The successful venture from the qualitative study contributed to a decision to initiate a second joint effort, that of testing newly developed instruments to measure fatigue from the three perspectives. The items for these instruments were derived from the qualitative data from the focus group sessions.

CONCLUSION

Through selected examples, strategies for forming, developing, and maintaining different types of teams (from same discipline, same site to multidisciplinary, multisite) that are involved in qualitative research endeavors have been delineated. Particular attention has been given to strategies for selecting team members, study sites, the study focus, and the research methodology and to the actions that foster team efforts and contribute to a stronger and more credible research product or program. The examples emphasize the need for team members to seriously commit time, energy, and ideas to the team, as well as to the research, as "team" and "research" for qualitative studies are inextricably bound.

REFERENCES

Adler, P. A., & Adler, P. (1987). *Membership roles in field research.* Newbury Park, CA: Sage.

Allen, K. R., & Walker, A. J. (1992). A feminist analysis of interviews with elderly mothers and their daughters. In J. F. Gilgun, K. Daly, & G. Handel (Eds.), *Qualitative methods in family research* (pp. 198-214). Newbury Park, CA: Sage.

Birenbaum, L., Hinds, P., & Clarke-Steffen, L. (1995). Multisite qualitative nursing research in pediatric oncology. *Journal of Pediatric Oncology Nursing, 12,* 135-139.

Denzin, N. (1989). *The research act: A theoretical introduction to sociological methods* (3rd ed.; pp. 234-239). Englewood Cliffs, NJ: Prentice Hall.

Denzin, N. (1989). *The research act: A theoretical introduction to sociological methods* (3rd ed.; pp. 234-239). Englewood Cliffs, NJ: Prentice Hall.

Erickson, K., & Stull, D. (1998). *Doing team ethnography: Warnings and advice.* Thousand Oaks, CA: Sage.

Gates, M. F., & Lackey, N. R. (1998). Youngsters caring for adults with cancer. *Image: Journal of Nursing Scholarship, 20,* 11-15.

Gates, M. F., Lackey, N. R., & Brown, G. (1996). *Black women's lived/caring experiences with breast cancer: Final report.* Memphis, TN: Oncology Nursing Foundation.

Grady, K. E. & Wallston, B. S. (1988). *Research in health care settings.* Newbury Park, CA: Sage.

Hinds, P., Birenbaum, L., Clarke-Steffen, L., Quargnenti, A., Kreissman, S., Kazak, A., Meyer, W., Pratt, C., Mulhern, R., & Wiliams, J. (1996). Coming to terms: Parents' response to a first cancer recurrence. *Nursing Research 45,* 148-153.

Hinds, P. S., Hockenberry-Eaton, M., Quargnenti, A., May, M., Burleson, C., Gilger, E., Randall, E., & O'Neill, J. (1999). Fatigue in 7- to 12-year-old patients with cancer from the staff perspective: An exploratory study. *Oncology Nursing Forum, 16,* 37-45.

Hockenberry-Eaton, M., Hinds, P., Alcoser, P., Brace-O'Neil, J., Euell, K., Howard, V., Gattuso, J., & Taylor, J. (1998). Fatigue in children and adolescents with cancer. *Journal of Pediatric Oncology Nursing, 15,* 172-182.

Krippendorff, K. (1980). *Content analysis: An introduction to its methodology.* Beverly Hills, CA: Sage.

Lackey, N. R., & Gates, M. F. (1994). *Family needs study: Final report.* Memphis, TN: Sigma Theta Tau Beta Chapter-At-Large.

Lackey, N. R., & Gates, M. F. (1997). Combining the analyses of three qualitative data sets in studying young caregivers. *Journal of Advanced Nursing, 26,* 664-671.

Lincoln, Y., & Guba, E. (1985). *Naturalistic inquiry.* Beverly Hills, CA: Sage.

Pickett, M., Brennan, A. M. W., Greenberg, H. S., Licht, L., & Worrell, J. D. (1994). Use of debriefing techniques to prevent compassion fatigue in research teams. *Nursing Research, 43,* 250-252.

Tripp-Reimer, T., Sorofman, B., Peters, J., & Waterman, J. E. (1994). Research teams: Possibilities and pitfalls in collaborative qualitative research. In J. M. Morse (Ed.), *Critical issues in qualitative research methods* (pp. 318-331). Thousand Oaks, CA: Sage.

10

On Being Part of the Audience

Richard L. Ochberg

The editors of this volume have asked us to discuss our personal reactions to doing interview research; this is a discussion that rarely finds its way into print. I must confess that much as I want to hear what others have to say, the invitation makes me uneasy. I am a clinical psychologist; I was taught that if our clients provoke any sort of reaction from us—if they arouse our pity, envy, lust, or even our admiration—we may be less able to listen attentively to them. I still believe this—and I believe that we have to listen dispassionately to our research informants as well.

At the same time, it seems obvious that both our clients and our research informants frequently do provoke us in one way or another—and that doing so may be the point of the stories that they tell us. A story is told for the purpose of affecting its audience; therefore, to see what narrators are up to, we must examine the effect that they are trying to create. Of course, what matters is not the way narrators affect academic interviewers but rather the audiences in their real lives: their families, friends, neighbors, employers, and so on. Nevertheless, we interviewers can report, firsthand, how our informants affected us; this may be a useful point of departure.[1]

The idea of paying attention to how life stories affect audiences is by no means novel. For example, Susan Harding (1992) describes how an informant of hers—a fundamentalist minister—tried to convert her by recounting a particularly tragic event in his own life. On a much broader stage, Erikson (1950, 1975) suggested that both Hitler and Gandhi used their autobiographies to enlist the support of their followers. Linde (1993) points out that we all tell each other life stories all the time—and that these exchanges regulate our intimacy. Last, many psychotherapists assume that our clients tell us stories not merely to fill us in on events outside the office but to create a relationship with us. Therefore, we continually ask our clients, "What does it mean for you to be telling me this story now?"

In this essay, I would like to propose a variation on our usual understanding of how storytellers address their audiences. Usually, we assume that they try to make themselves understood. This seems logical: If one's self-image depends on how others react, it seems natural that narrators would want their audiences to understand and agree with them. Therefore, most storytellers emphasize only those experiences and reasons that their audiences find plausible (Rosenwald & Wiersma, 1983; Tolman, 1991), they tell their stories in genres that their audiences are likely to recognize (Harding, 1992; Modell, 1992), and they explain away whatever their audiences might find inappropriate (Linde, 1993).

There is, however, another possibility, suggested by the model of psychotherapy. In therapy, as in interview research, one person tells another a life story; ostensibly, our clients, like research informants, are trying to make themselves understood. Most therapists, however, recognize that their clients may actually be far more ambivalent. Their lives have led them to regard others with suspicion: Any audience may prove disinterested, jealous, incompetent, or vengeful. To speak too openly is to risk having one's words turned against one. Therefore, clients often look for ways to elude their therapists' understanding; they maneuver the interview situation so that their therapists—rather than they themselves —can be put in the wrong. In fact, it is often said that the real focus of therapy is not exactly the story that clients tell but the continual repair of whatever mistrust has made narration difficult.

Here, I want to see whether we can extend the therapeutic model of dialogue to the research interview. Many of our informants have their own reasons to doubt our good intentions. Therefore, the stories that they tell us are not wholly a way of making connections; they are also a way of keeping us at bay. Recognizing this would, I think, extend our understanding of how personal narration works.

Before turning to cases, I want to acknowledge that this approach to interviews is not how I started out. I began interviewing people about their careers, rather than asking them to fill out questionnaires, because this seemed more likely to lead to detailed and vivid descriptions. At that time (25 years ago), I was interested exclusively in the substance of their stories, not their rhetorical strategies. Now, however, I see a connection between what I hoped to hear about careers and my current view of narrative interpretation.

I have been strongly influenced by Erikson, who pointed out that identity is, in part, interpersonal. We know ourselves—maybe we even are ourselves—by way of how we matter to others. Applying this idea to vocational identity, I imagined that careers might be (among many other things) a way of putting ourselves on a public stage: Depending on how our audiences respond to us, we may deem ourselves competent, virtuous, lovable—or not. To give a popular phrase a punning, psychodynamic meaning, a career might be a way to "make something of oneself." Of course, I assumed that the self-images that narrators see reflected in the eyes of an audience matter because of the life historical resonances they evoke.

Today, I see a connection between this Eriksonian view of vocational identity and a particular way of regarding life stories. By paying attention to how stories affect audiences—and what this means to narrators—we also see how selves are made through other kinds of public performances, such as careers.

I am going to focus on a man I call Al Silver, who I interviewed for a study of middle-aged businessmen (Ochberg, 1992, 1996). Given that this is a discussion of audience response, it may help to describe my first impression. Al was a singularly difficult man to interview. Of course, it is always hard getting started in this business. We show up on a stranger's doorstep—armed with a tape recorder, no less—and start asking the sort of invasive questions that even one's closer friends avoid. Usually, however, we manage to forge some sort of alliance with our informants: We promise to take them seriously and to try to see their points of view. On this basis, we generally stumble past the first awkward moments and launch ourselves on what is, at least initially, a collaborative venture. Al was uniquely antagonistic to this collaboration.

He failed to arrive for our first scheduled meeting and offered no apology. He began our first interview by telling me how contemptuous he was of professional academics. "There is a pervading sense of superiority, which I suppose I was once guilty of myself. It seems to be based on job security and poor pay, which one has to compensate for one way or another." Later, I decided that his derision was directed as much toward his parents and his own previous career as it was toward me. In those first moments, however, I felt distinctly unwelcome. This may also have had something to do with his bored, truculent tone or the fact that he kept interrupting our conversation to make phone calls. Eventually, I turned off the tape recorder and offered to cancel the whole engagement—something I have never done with anyone else. Somehow, we agreed to continue, and by the end of the evening, Al had decided that we were *landsmen:* big-city East Coasters marooned in a Midwest village, cultural sophisticates, Jewish liberals, and loyal sons. He took me upstairs to see a portrait of his father—further, that is, into the private territory of his home than I am usually invited.

Eventually, I saw that this mixture of pushing me away and inviting me in was typical of Al. The stories that he told about himself had much the same effect as his behavior: They made him seem alternately attractive and thoroughly dislik-able. Furthermore, he had apparently done the same thing with others through-out his life: He had been in alternate moments (maybe even the same moment) a loyal disciple and a boorish rebel. Perhaps most interesting was the way he de-scribed one employer who, he felt, may have understood him. Al sounded genu-inely touched by this man—for a sentence or two—then he quickly discredited his boss's insight, thereby rekindling the possibility that he had been misunder-stood after all. Now, I need to say this carefully. I do not think that Al really hopes to be misunderstood; in fact, when he is, he becomes angry. More exactly, Al presents himself in such a way that all understanding is forever suspect. This seems important to him. The point seems to be that whatever impression one forms of Al might be wrong; his audience might always turn out to have misjudged him. This, in turn, allows him to escape a greater danger: that he will let down his guard, turn into the sort of person that his audience might under-stand—and thereby lose himself.

At the time that I interviewed him, Al was 41; for the past 6 years, he had sold real estate. This was a sharp departure from both the academic career that he had hoped to pursue when he started graduate school in American history and his 3 years in publishing.

Selling real estate was also a long way from his parents' careers: His father was an art historian and a musicologist, his mother, a professor of English. Al himself emphasized the contrast between his current life and the refined world in which he was raised. Both of his parents were sensitive connoisseurs of books, music, and art. His mother, he said, "was a very sensitive, intense woman." He told admiring stories about his father that border on the fantastic.

> He could look at a print and tell you if the color was right. Had he never seen the original, he would tell you if the color was right or wrong. . . . I watched him iden-tify a piece of music he had never heard. He said, "It's got to be this." He once drove a music contest off the air: He won it every day for four weeks. Godawful ob-scure music, snippets.

Refinement, however, was not simply a matter of cultural sophistication; it was a whole ensemble of values and style. For example, both of his parents were politically committed: members of the Communist Part in the era when Joe McCarthy made that choice unhealthy. They were disdainful of money. They were restrained in their appetites and (so they at least claimed) their emotions. Both parents, Al said, were well-known and admired in the intellectual circles in which they moved, "genuinely respected and humble people."

In contrast, the picture that Al drew of himself—or at least one of his self-portraits—is the very antithesis of everything his parents valued. For example, "I was expected to be a good student and I hated the stuff, expected to be diligent and save every nickel and I never saved a Goddamned penny." These days, "Real estate allows me to work as hard as I want and make as much as I want. I spend every bloody penny of it, frankly."

As a child, he was punished for being too aggressive—fighting with his sister, with whom he said, "there was bitter competition." In real estate, however,

I could sell anything to anyone, and they loved me for it. I really loved the work; it was legitimized aggression. I got paid for what I used to get kicked in the ass for: being aggressive and stating my opinions.

His parents were willing to put their political values on the line. At one time, Al shared their commitment, but those days are long gone:

I don't get the same emotional reward that I used to, crusading for every stray dog or small social issue that I could get hot under the collar about. . . . In college, my hair was halfway down my back and I wore a lot of funny clothes. I spent a lot of time marching up and down in front of Kroger's, worrying about the United Farm Workers; I went to DC [to protest Vietnam], and frankly, on both of those issues, I would do them again if called upon. But [now] I have more personal goals: I am de-voted to career development.

So far, Al's story seems familiar enough. He was raised to be one sort of per-son, but he rejected his parents' life style and forged his own. Selling real estate lets him stick a thumb in the eye of those cultural pretenders who let him down long ago. At this point, however, the picture gets more complicated. Through a dozen small vignettes, Al warns us that things are not quite what they seem.

First of all, it turns out on closer inspection that supposedly refined people are not without their faults. His parents may have been widely admired in their culti-vated circle, but they had a stormy marriage. As a child, Al did not know what the fights were about, he could only report what his mother told him, years later: that her husband mistreated her and that he was infuriatingly stingy. Al continued,

He was not a good father to me. In my early years he was critical and bad tempered. I never saw him much and when I did there was a lot of emotion involved, rarely any of it any good. I was afraid of him. I wasn't beaten but chased. I had all the signs of an emotionally abused child: bed wetter into my early years, asthma, hay fever, extreme tension, lack of attentiveness.

His mother may have been "sensitive," but she was also

a very dour woman, sour even. She came out of childhood with the name Mary Sunshine, and the corner candy store operator called her Bubbles. Well, she was old sour puss herself. [The nicknames, Al explained, were mocking.] Her hair was always pulled back. She never wore fancy clothes, or good clothes. Never treated herself as female.

As for his sister:

> It is funny, because in many ways she is a very tender woman, very sensitive. She has an eye for shape and form; very expressive. It is a very energetic part of her. . . . [However], there is no warmth to her at all. Cold as ice. Her warmth is superficial.

Not too surprisingly, Al's critique of his family extends to other significant players in his life whose superficial gentility masks a darker underside. His current boss, Spencer Ames, seems to be a gentleman, who naturally regards Al with well-bred distaste.

> He respects me, but only as an employee. I have been working there six years. In that time, in most other companies, there would have been a closer business relationship. I have no more progress with him or trust than the day I started.
> He is always the gentleman—not one of my stronger points. I offend a lot of people. Someone once referred to me as a "heavy." To me, that's a compliment; to Spencer, that would be an offense.
> He takes offense at things he considers to be social ungraces . . . at my willingness to be critical of others, at my brashness. Just emotionally he is offended by the intense way I relate to people personally.

If Al's bluntly aggressive and materialistic approach to real estate reenacts his defiant childhood, Spencer's cultivated disapproval echoes that of Al's refined parents.

Yet it turns out, at least according to Al, that Spencer has the usual faults of so-called gentlefolk.

> He is fond of everyone and close to no one. He is a ferocious tennis player; he can knock the shit out of someone half his age, but always, very clean. Tennis is a gentleman's game. You never hear an off-color comment or a dirty word from Spencer. Never a raised voice; you rarely see him frustrated or angry.
> Spencer does not have a good sense of the needs and expectations of the people who work for him. . . . It is reflected in his home life. His wife has reported to me with some pain that he wasn't much of a father. He found it difficult to relate to the needs of his daughters. He didn't see the connection between them and him, didn't take them very close into his heart. He ran them the way he runs business. Waitresses, daughters, they are all the same. A very distant man, covered up by this gentle, quiet demeanor.

Last, in explaining how he decided to go to graduate school, Al offered this curious description. Reading through an old songbook, he came upon a Shaker dirge that so moved him that he became obsessed with American history.

> The music itself was terribly moving, and it kindled an interest that I'd had all along in community building. Not because I think [the Shakers] are great; I think they are a bunch of idiots, frankly. They are a pretty rough bunch toward each other. They are rigid and demanding, a rather humorless group.

Each of these descriptions makes the same argument. All of these characters are sensitive about impersonal things (art, music, public decorum), but they are cold and sometimes brutal toward each other. His sister is "emotional" about art but "cold as ice" toward people. Spencer will not swear on a tennis court, but he is a "ferocious" player who will "knock the shit out of an opponent," and he treats his daughters like employees. The Shakers may have created terribly moving music but they were "a pretty rough bunch" toward each other. Furthermore, like Al's mother, the Shakers sound dour, sexless, and self-abnegating.

There is an interesting counterpart to this description. If supposedly refined people turn out, on closer inspection, to be less admirable than they first seem, Al himself turns out to have his own half-hidden virtues.

For example, real estate has a reputation for attracting cutthroat salesmen. However, Al said,

> I really see myself as a counselor. Oddly, or not oddly at all, I have always had very strong relations with the academic community, with people who don't respond well to the used-car types. I deal with a billion divorcees, widows . . . and I have a very strong influence within that kind of community.

Furthermore, he feels that money is not really his goal.

> I am living with the belief that I am supposed to be challenged at all times. That money is not a very good goal, it is a tool to something else, but that the real goal in life is some kind of development and challenge.

Although Al has a keen eye for academic pretension, and although he described himself as "an East Coast snob from the word go," it turns out that he is an amateur scholar of the small, Midwestern town in which he has landed. He is an avid collector of ancient city directories and plat books, the old county records that document who owned parcels of land generations ago. He knows the history of tiny local towns and manufacturing concerns. Nor does he confine himself to documents:

> I owned a Goddamned grist mill in Waterloo before I gave it back to the guy I bought it from. [RO: Why did you buy it?] Fucked if I know. I lost a bundle on it. I couldn't restore it. It was a good idea, I thought. I liked the big old sifters, and the wooden beams. . . . We are talking about how people organized their lives. A mill or a factory is simply an organization of people. Somebody had to decide to build miniature motor parts and hire other people, and they built a community around it.

There is, clearly, a discrepancy between the images that Al presents us. At first glance, he is a Philistine; on closer examination, he is a truer gentleman than those who criticize him. Suppose that we now ask, What sort of impression does Al want us to have of him? One possibility is that he wants us to see him as a complex man: aggressive, materialistic, self-centered—and yet for all that, more profoundly cultured, caring, and civic minded than those who presume to judge him. I think that this is, in fact, the way Al sees himself. However, I also think that what Al wants from us may be more complicated—he (partly) wants us to misunderstand him—and this is one reason that he presents himself in so contradictory a fashion. I realize that this must seem unlikely; here is my evidence.

Al apparently has a history of making it difficult for audiences to understand him. Here, for example, he describes his career as a student.

> I was the world's worst scholar. I hated high school and elementary school. I didn't apply myself, I wasn't interested in what I was studying. I got out of high school by the very skin of my teeth. Oddly, I never missed a day of school past the eighth grade. And I also was never there on time, never raised my hand and never did any work.

In his senior year, he applied to only one college, Columbia, and was rejected. Then (as Al tells the story), the admissions office received his SAT scores—all in the 700's—and invited him for an interview. "Which I did the next day. Just caught a train, walked in, and said, 'Here I am: Interview me.' And I was accepted 2 days later."

In a strikingly similar anecdote, he describes the man who hired him for his first job selling real estate.

> He was very generous of himself, he gave me a lot. When he hired me, I had hair halfway down my back; I wore blue jeans and smoked cigars. My only vehicle was a truck, and a battered up one at that. I wouldn't have hired me on a bet. Not only [did he hire me] he gave a shit whether I succeeded: Told me when I was doing good and chewed me out when I made mistakes; always with real affection.

Each of these vignettes makes the same point. To any casual observer, Al must have seemed a bad-natured, untalented kid who deserved little consideration. However, a more attentive observer would have seen the deeper truth. His high school teachers were probably irritated by his horrible grades and defiant manner, but they should have noticed his perfect attendance. The admissions committee at Columbia might have rejected him for his grades and his ill-mannered approach ("Here I am: Interview me"); instead, they were swayed by his Board scores. His first boss could have been dismayed by Al's haircut and cigars, or he might have noticed that Al's vita promised more than his uncouth appearance.

These three vignettes turn the tables on us. Up to this point, we have assumed that Al is trying to justify his life. This is a standard idea in narrative interpretation, and Al has more explaining to do than most people; after all, he has become the antithesis of everything he was brought up to admire. Suddenly, we realize that Al is not the only one on trial; his audiences are, too. The issue is no longer simply, what sort of man is Al? but, how closely has anyone—his teachers, his employers, or you and I—been paying attention?

The most interesting thing about the last anecdote is the way it ended. Eventually, I asked Al what hidden talent his first employer might have seen in him. He replied,

> I don't know that he saw anything at first. I don't know if he had the brains to know a good agent from a bad one. It was no great compliment that he took me; I was scuzzier than most. He hired a lot of well-dressed bums, most had 2 years [junior college] if that, or 37 years of failure behind them. Now, if you really sat down and profiled me, I wasn't likely to fail in quite the same way, but I don't think he understood that.

What are to make of this last passage? If, as our interpretive theories tell us, the point of self-presentation is to be understood, then Al seems to have gone out of his way to snatch yet another defeat from the jaws of victory. Here, it would seem, is the one good man in Al's story: Someone who cared enough to understand Al's promise no matter how unpromising he first appeared. Yet Al's conclusion denies himself even this one connection: His boss was a drunken fool who probably did not understand Al at all. "Heart as big as the world, probably a liver to match it. Big ideas, small capacity to follow through on them." Al's gloss on his own history seems decidedly peculiar—unless, of course, being understandable is, for him, the greatest danger of all.

I think that Al is trying to accomplish several things by making himself difficult to understand. First of all, he is testing his audience: Do they care enough to pay attention? As we have heard, Al feels that he was unfairly criticized: for fighting with his sister, doing poorly in school, being a spendthrift. Furthermore,

Al suggested that his parents were so consumed by their war with each other that they paid little attention to his distress. For example,

> The popular dogs of the day were very assertive: boxers and high strung poodles. A whole bunch of them, and I was always a paperboy. I got bit in my work frequently. Nobody thought those dogs were biting kids. You were afraid of them and nobody did anything about it.

Now of course, I do not think that being bitten was the formative trauma in Al's life; however, I think that it is no accident that he recounts this story. The point of this recollection is not the event in itself but the moral: People who should have been paying attention were not.

In addition to testing his audience, Al's difficult self-presentation preserves a quality that he values in himself: his defiant willfulness. Here, two passages suggest what Al might lose were he easier to understand.

Earlier, we heard that Al took up American history because he was smitten with the Shakers; however, his admiration was distinctly mixed. The Shakers may have written beautiful music, but they were also (like Al's parents or Spencer) a brutal, humorless lot. It turns out that Al had other objections to them.

> There was something about the emotionalism of [the music] that I found appealing, though I can't come to terms with their rather pathetic philosophy, which was terribly humble. I think in many regards they were very much at peace with themselves. Perhaps it was a sense that I don't have about myself—I am not at peace with myself. Certainly in joining the community, they gave up all ambition. I have a great fondness for tranquility that I don't have. I couldn't live with it either, to be honest. No way in hell. Fucking or no fucking [the Shakers were celibate], that is not the weakness. The weakness is that they had no will, and I've got plenty.

Al's description of the Shakers is curiously similar to a daydream that he sometimes entertains about his future. He hopes that Spencer will make him a partner—but he knows that this is unlikely. If things do not work out with Spencer, Al imagines retiring to a small town on the Navajo reservation in New Mexico.

> Working in Chinle, or some other little speck on the map. Perhaps writing, which I have never attempted, perhaps simple good deeds, if you will. A committed and dedicated life. That's one of the directions I keep looking; one of a charitable or rather a self-sacrificing nature.

I do not for a moment imagine that this daydream is a serious possibility; nevertheless, I find the imagery suggestive. Writing, doing good deeds, commitment, dedication: This is the life his parents might have admired. The problem, however, is suggested by the way Al amends his description: "A charitable, *or rather a self-sacrificing nature.*" The phrase reminds us of what he said about the Shakers: Terribly humble, pathetic people—who in joining a community of virtue gave up all ambition and will.

In other words, to become the sort of man his parents would have understood and admired, Al would have to be not only scholarly, civic minded, and charitable, but, above all, self-abnegating. He half-believes that they were right and that he might yet resurrect these abandoned virtues in himself. Yet to do so would be to abandon his "will," to become, like the Shakers, "pathetic." Ever since he was a child, he has met his parents' disapproval with defiance; he is not about to stop now.

With this in mind, we can now see why Al seems deliberately to confound his audiences. Someone with a different personality might be happy to feel understood; however, too much of Al's life has been energized by his resentment: This demands continual replenishment. Were Al to make it easy for anyone to approve of him, were he even to admit that someone along the line did approve and that this touched him, he would risk surrendering his defiant willfulness. So, despite the fact that Al (partly) wants to be recognized as cultured and civic minded, he'll be damned before he makes this recognition easy or admits that it matters to him.

CONCLUSION

At the start of this discussion, I suggested two ideas. First, the stories that people tell about themselves—whether in research, psychotherapy, or daily life—affect their relationship with whoever is listening. For example, narrators do not simply tell us that they have been admired (or belittled, or misunderstood, or seduced and abandoned) all their lives. In addition, they tell us their stories in some characteristic style: amusingly, sarcastically, angrily, provokingly, suspiciously, seductively, and so on. Each of these styles establishes a particular rapport between them and us; it turns us into partners in their private drama; this in turn reconfirms the narrator's self-understanding. Therefore, to see what a life story means, we have to see what effect the speaker is trying to create. Although this way of paying attention to personal accounts is not yet routine in interview research, it is becoming more common.

The second and more controversial idea is that narrators may not expect—or even want—their audiences to understand them in the same way that they understand themselves. At first glance, this may seem implausible.

For example, Linde (1993, p. 12) suggests that the point of a life story is to create "coherence." By this, she means that a story creates a certain kind of sense and that the person to whom it is told must recognize and be persuaded by the sort of sense that the story makes. "The speaker works to construct a text whose coherence can be appreciated, and at the same time the addressee works to reach some understanding of it as a coherent text." Linde acknowledges that, "the coherent text that the addressee constructs may not, of course, be the same as the text that the speaker believes was constructed." However—and this is the essential point—"if [the gap] becomes very large, further negotiation about the meaning of the text may be necessary."

At first glance, Linde seems to be making much the same point that I have tried to emphasize. Our sense of ourselves depends on our experience of how others understand us. However, I do not think that our sense of ourselves necessarily depends on others seeing us *the same way* that we see ourselves. In fact, just the opposite may be the case. Our sense of who we are may depend on feeling that others see us differently than we see ourselves. We may, for example, cherish the idea that we are keeping a secret (Ochberg, 1994), or—as in Al's case—that we are too complicated for any but the most attentive audience to comprehend (compare Erikson, 1946).[2]

The interpretive approach that I am advocating draws together something that we already know about both artistic expression and lives. In any field of art, we can point to examples whose effect depends on their resistance to facile apprehension. *Ulysses,* for example, would not be clearer were it written by Hemingway rather than Joyce; instead, it would be something altogether different. Our difficulty in grasping *Ulysses* is intrinsic to our experience of it. The same goes for Magritte's image of a pipe and its deliberately confounding subtitle, "Ceci n'est pas une pipe."

In an analogous fashion, we all know any number of people who seem distinctly ambivalent about being understood. Such people may feel distrustful: They want to feel connected to others, yet they suspect that others may be indifferent or dangerous. For anyone who doubts the perfect goodwill of their audience, telling a transparently open life story may seem foolish: To do so might leave one open to contempt or betrayal. If, instead, the goal is to create relationships that are only partially open, one must tell stories that are semi-opaque. Such stories must engage an audience yet keep that audience at a distance. Telling a story in this manner—and thereby creating a guarded or contested relationship with one's listener—in turn confirms a particular sense of self. (In a study of choreographers, Evans [1992] makes much the same point about the psychological uses of resisting one's audience.)

Throughout this discussion, I have had in the back of my mind a visual analogy. There is a well-known design that represents either a Greek vase or two faces turned toward each other, depending on what one takes to be the foreground and background. What makes this design interesting is, of course, not its literal subject matter—the faces or the vase—but the effect that it has on us.

Once we realize that there are two possible perceptions, we cannot be content with seeing one or the other: We try to see both at once. However, this is impossible, the two images are mutually exclusive, we can never see two faces *and* a vase at the same time. This leaves us with a curious experience of the image and of ourselves. Our experience is not that of seeing two faces or a vase—and certainly not of seeing both together—but rather of our own inability to see what we know is there. No matter which image we see, we are partly wrong, if also—but less significantly—partly right.

I have been trying to say something similar about Al's depiction of himself. Some of the things that Al says about himself (and does) reconnect him to his artistic, scholarly, and civic-minded parents. At the same time, Al suspects that cultivated folks disapprove of him, and he feels that he would lose his "will" if he made himself more acceptable. Therefore, he says and does other things that make him seem boorish. Like the design, there is no easy way to synthesize these opposite impressions; taken together, they make Al difficult to read. Al forces us to see him first one way and then the other; no matter what we decide about him, it seems, a moment later, that we have misconstrued him. His self-depiction challenges us, it unsettles us, it puts us forever in the wrong—and this is its point. Al, like the design, continually confounds an audience that he suspects does not have his interests at heart instead of weakly acquiescing with what others expect. For Al, like the ambiguous design, the point is not to create a meeting of the minds but an interpretive struggle.

Suppose we agree that some informants—how many, we cannot say—have reservations about being too easily understood. They mistrust their would-be understanders, or they fear losing some quality in themselves if they are too readily grasped. Where does this leave us—as researchers or therapists?

Looking at the matter naively, we may be inclined to wish that their suspicion could be allayed. Surely (we might imagine), we would hear their stories more clearly if only their relationship with us did not get in the way. This, however, is a mistake. The stories our informants tell us and their relationship with us are two sides of the same coin: The meaning of the story is inseparable from its effect on the listener.

Well then, (one might continue), we might at least try to make this relationship as smooth as possible. Surely, the story will be purest and most detailed if our informants can speak without mistrusting us. This too is a mistake. We would not understand Al better if his story did not set us up to misjudge him; instead, we would not understand him at all—because he would no longer be himself.

Personality is (among many other things) the particular way that each of us recreates and attempts to overcome whatever dangers matter to us. We do not become more fully ourselves in the absence of these (protectively constructed) dangers; instead—were such a thing possible—we would no longer be ourselves at all. Therefore, not only is it inevitable that our informants struggle against us, this struggle may be essential to their self-creation—and to our appreciation of them. To see how narrators struggle with their audiences—pushing them away and pulling them closer, inviting understanding and disparaging it—is to see more of the complexity in both life stories and lives.

NOTES

1. Now that I have finished this essay, I see that I might well have gone in a different direction. Rather than focus on what our personal experience teaches us about our informants, we might examine what we learn about ourselves. We might put the matter in terms of a familiar methodological point: It only occurs to us to interpret our informants' stories when we realize that they are trying to make a different kind of sense than any that we anticipated (explaining a moral decision in terms of care instead of justice, for example). To understand them is to illuminate simultaneously what they—we—take for granted; this makes every study partly a voyage of self-discovery; what we learn about ourselves may be as interesting as anything else. I take this idea seriously; however, it is not the direction I will pursue here.

2. Erikson is not usually thought of as a narratologist, yet there is a striking parallel between his account of identity and current theories of life stories. Erikson (1946) said, "The conscious feeling of having a personal identity is based on two simultaneous observations: the immediate perception of one's self-sameness and continuity in time; and the simultaneous perception of the fact that others recognize one's self-sameness and continuity" (p. 365). Life stories create both sides of this experience. First, life stories create a conviction of personal continuity—"self-sameness"—out of what one might otherwise experience as randomly discordant episodes (Cohler, 1988; Linde, 1993; Mishler, 1992). In addition, by framing their stories in recognizable genres, narrators win the ratification of their audiences (Harding, 1992; Modell, 1992). That is: personal narratives matter because they fashion identity. Of course, the interesting thing about Erikson is that he recognized the limits of identity—if only as a passing phase. Some young people need to repudiate what others expect of them to feel more certain of having made their own choices: Erikson referred to this option as a "negative identity," which might be assumed in a safely temporary moratorium. In describing this strategy—we might call it "identity resistance"—Erikson was far more sensitive to the potential struggle between would-be selves and audiences than most contemporary narratologists have been.

REFERENCES

Cohler, B. (1988). The human studies and the life history: The Social Service Review lecture. *Social Service Review, 62*(4), 552-575.
Erikson, E. (1946). Ego development and historical change. *The Psychoanalytic Study of the Child, 2,* 359-396.
Erikson, E. (1950). *Childhood and society.* New York: Norton.

Erikson, E. (1975). *Life history and the historical moment.* New York: Norton.

Evans, J. (1992). Language and the body: Communication and identity formation in choreography. In G. Rosenwald & R. Ochberg (Eds.), *Storied lives* (pp. 95-107). New Haven, CT: Yale University Press.

Harding, S. (1992). The afterlife of stories: Genesis of a man of God. In G. Rosenwald & R. Ochberg (Eds.), *Storied lives* (pp. 60-75). New Haven, CT: Yale University Press.

Linde, C. (1993). *Life stories: The creation of coherence.* New York: Oxford University Press.

Mishler, E. (1992). Work, identity, and narrative. In G. Rosenwald & R. Ochberg (Eds.), *Storied lives* (pp. 21-40). New Haven, CT: Yale University Press.

Modell, J. (1992). How do you introduce yourself as a childless mother? In G. Rosenwald & R. Ochberg (Eds.), *Storied lives* (pp. 76-94). New Haven, CT: Yale University Press.

Ochberg, R. (1992). Patterns of unhappiness in men's careers. In R. Young & A. Collin (Eds.), *Interpreting career* (pp. 98-116). Westport, CT: Praeger.

Ochberg, R. (1994). Life stories and storied lives. In A. Lieblich & R. Josselson (Eds.), *The narrative study of lives, 2* (pp. 113-144). Thousand Oaks, CA: Sage.

Ochberg, R. (1996). Interpreting life stories. In A. Lieblich & R. Josselson (Eds.), *The narrative study of lives, 4* (pp. 97-113). Thousand Oaks, CA: Sage.

Rosenwald, G. C., & Wiersma, J. (1983). Women, career changes, and the new self. *Psychiatry, 46,* 213-229.

Tolman, D. (1991). Adolescent girls, women, and sexuality: Discerning dilemmas of desire. In C. Gilligan, A. Rogers, & D. Tolman (Eds.), *Women, girls, and psychotherapy.* New York: Harrington Park.

PART 3

Reporting the Researcher Experience

11

The Research Experience as Described in Published Reports

Susan Diemert Moch

If the researcher experience troubles us as it does, and if the researcher experience is often included in presentations at research conferences, research methods seminars, and in conversations with research colleagues, why is evidence of the researcher experience so limited in published works? This chapter provides an overview of published material on the researcher experience.

We have often discussed the researcher experience with each other and with other colleagues. We have heard researchers speak of the researcher's experience in presentations at research conferences. We have frequently wondered why talking about the researcher experience is acceptable but writing about the experience and getting the researcher experience accepted for publication is unlikely. Not talking about the researcher experience may further exacerbate denial of the researcher experience for researchers and publishers. Maybe if the researcher is purposefully left out of the research report, the research can seem more "objective" and "true."

I wondered if reviewers for a manuscript I submitted to a major nursing journal years ago wished to deny the existence of the researcher experience. The manuscript, titled "Incorporating the Researcher Experience Into Nursing Research Reporting," was rejected. One reviewer wrote across the front page of the manuscript in bold, capital letters, "NO OBJECTIVITY." Such a reproach was probably considered the ultimate in criticism by the reviewer, but "no objectivity" was precisely the point I was trying to make in the manuscript. Including the researcher experience in research reporting may call into question the objectivity rule of science. Insistence on the objectivity rule in research journals may be the reason scientific journals do not include the researcher experience.

Now, however, more researchers acknowledge the difficulty with allegiance to objectivity. Research methodologists, Reinharz (1992), Moustakas (1990), and Paterson and Zderad (1976) have advocated for use of the researcher experience in experiential analysis, heuristic research, and phenomenological nursology, respectively. In addition, anthropologist Ruth Behar (1993) and sociologist Susan Krieger (1991) have led efforts to demonstrate how the research experience can be included in research reporting. Behar (1993) and Krieger (1991) argue that the researcher experience is present, no matter how much researchers try to ignore the presence of the researcher within the research report. In fact, reporting holistic finding demands the inclusion of the researcher experience. Krieger (1991, 1996) and Behar (1993, 1996) share reflections about what to do with the researcher experience in their books, as indicated in the following section.

RESEARCH EXPERIENCES
SHARED IN BOOKS

Books offer great freedom in talking about the researcher experience. To publish in book form, authors need not convince traditional peer reviewers that the researcher experience is important to the research report. Through book form, authors have the liberty and often the space to share the researcher experience. With books, rather than in journals, specific space allocation is not usually an issue. Often, because qualitative research reports require more space for reporting than the more traditional, quantitative research reports, the research experience is omitted. Also, guidelines for reporting research in journals are usually much more stringent than for books. A section allocated for the researcher experience is rare in journals. So books also offer more flexibility than journals in reporting.

A 1979 book by Reinharz included the researcher experience. She discussed her involvement with research aimed at describing how families coped with intermittent rocket shelling. During the process of the research, she realized the importance of looking at her own reactions to her experience and the reported experience of others. She developed a process named *experiential analysis.* She said, "I cannot convey adequately the positive regard with which I viewed and felt enveloped by these families. . . . I came to cherish the families" (p. 312). Reinharz adds that when fieldworkers do not discuss their involvement with the families, it is perceived in the writing anyway. According to Reinharz, "the self can be used in research not only as an observer (as in participant observation), but also as a receiver and receptacle of experience that is to be explicated" (p. 241).

"Reclaiming Self-Awareness as a Source of Insight" is the title of a chapter by Reinharz (1979). Through the chapter, the author discusses experiential research and research-as-process. The author draws on philosophers such as Polanyi, Kierkegaard, and even Descartes, with his thoughts on a reflexive attitude, in discussing the need for self-awareness in research. Reinharz contends that "The act of discovering must be explained by the same rubric as that which is discovered" (p. 251). She further argues that "failure to include the scientist, the research process, and the reporting under the same set of contingencies has opened the way for unethical acts to be performed in the name of science" (p. 251). According to Reinharz, legitimizing self-awareness as a source of insight will "yield a fuller documentation of research processes and a greater awareness of the nature of social processes" (p. 256).

Moustakas's (1990) method of research, heuristic research, begins with the researcher's experience, and the experience remains central to the process of research. According to Moustakas (1990), "I begin the heuristic investigation with my own self-awareness and explicate that awareness with reference to a question or problem until an essential insight is achieved, one that will throw a beginning light onto a critical human experience" (p. 11). The heuristic process values the researcher's experience or the data "within" the researcher.

Phenomenological nursology, a method proposed by Paterson and Zderad in 1976, involves the researcher experience. Advocating a method that incorporates practice and research, Paterson and Zderad described a means by which the relationship of the researcher to the participant includes many of the same qualities inherent in the nurse-patient relationship. Use of expertise and intuition by the nurse in practice was similarly valued in the research practice method of phenomenological nursology. Phenomenological psychotherapy (Moustakas, 1995) includes many of the same synthesis characteristics for practice and research as described by Paterson and Zderad (1976).

In addition to writing a journal article that incorporates the researcher experience (Krieger, 1985), Krieger's two books explicate the essential nature of the researcher's voice. Initially in her research, Krieger (1985) described her striving to clearly articulate the participant's voice. However, in her later book, Krieger (1991) described a realization that she may not be able to describe another voice completely:

> I have come to feel more caught within myself. I am struck increasingly with the impossibility of getting outside my own skin. The more I try to grasp someone else's experience, the more I am impressed with how hard it is, how much beyond me that other experience really is. (p. 53)

Krieger's work (1991, 1996) demands a voice calling for inclusion of the researcher voice in a meaningful way. In *The Family Silver,* Krieger (1996) offers her own voice through a series of essays on her work. In an earlier book, *Social Science and the Self,* Krieger (1991) identified her struggle and her wish for more holistic strategies for reporting:

> If the social scientific task is to model the world faithfully, there is a need for strategies of interpretation that challenge blinders of conventional thinking, whether these blinders stem from old orthodoxies (e.g., positivism) or new ones (e.g., postmodernist relativism). The self can be used as a source of more truthful expression in the social science. (p. 55)

In *Translated Woman,* Behar (1993) describes her interview research over 3 years with a woman named Esperanza. The interviews are delivered in a new style that includes both testimonial novel and conversational oral storytelling. Behar (1996) says, "I've tried to keep Esperanza's voice at the center of the text, while also showing my efforts to hear and understand her, efforts that led me, ultimately, to my own voice" (pp. 13-14). Later, Behar says,

> In the last two parts of the book, my voice becomes more interwoven with my comadre's voice, and there is a switch in tone from my comadre telling me her historia to the forging between us of a meta-historia. (p. 14)

Behar (1993) recounts how researchers often make the subject vulnerable yet leave the researcher invulnerable through the telling of the story. She describes how Esperanza shared so much of herself, often in an indirect manner—especially in regard to sexuality. Behar questions the authority and distance often used by Western anthropologists in forthrightly telling these special intimacies held by the storyteller. Behar submits,

> We ask for revelations from others, but we reveal little or nothing of ourselves; we make others vulnerable, but we ourselves remain invulnerable. I've tried to do something a little different here. I stand revealed throughout the book as a character in the narrative, asking not always very cogent or useful questions of Esperanza. (p. 273)

In an edited book on research method, Bowers (1988), in talking about grounded theory, described the role of the researcher. She identified how the researcher becomes intentionally immersed in the world of the research subjects while maintaining some objectivity. In the book, she briefly described her process as a researcher in the data analysis of a study of adult caregivers and their aging parents. However, in a research report of the same research, published in a nursing journal, Bowers (1987) makes no mention of her personal process as a researcher.

Through a book chapter on being a phenomenological researcher, Bergum (1989) confidently discusses her process of personal and professional transformation in reporting her study of women's transformation to motherhood. Through her conversations with new mothers, Bergum describes her own reflection and identifies questions about life and developmental changes through her motherhood. She shared feeling vulnerable in giving her interpretations of the women's stories with them.

In a book for the general public (Moch, 1995), I reported on research with midlife women on the experience of breast cancer. Stories of the women in the research were organized by the themes from the research (Moch, 1990a). Short descriptions of each of the 20 women in the study were provided, as was a gift of understanding or lesson of life provided through each woman.

> Such lessons about life were good for me. I realized that now is the best time to nurture relationships—to share myself more with family, friends, and others in the world around me. I wondered if I, too, could learn to become more perceptive through the wisdom of these women. I was interviewing my teachers and they were teaching me to slow down, reflect on my life, and open the boundaries dividing me from the world. (Moch, 1995, p. 131)

In the Field: Readings on the Field Research Experience, a book edited by Smith and Kornblum (1996), includes discussions by experienced researchers on topics such as gaining entry, building relationships, maintaining objectivity, and the observer's role in ethnography. The editors' intent was to share personal accounts "to give students and other readers a taste of what it is really like to conduct research 'in the field' " (p. v). According to the authors, the researcher's experience can profoundly affect the researcher. But the editors do not discuss how the researcher experience could then affect the research findings or the outcome of the research.

RESEARCH EXPERIENCES IN NURSING JOURNALS

Despite longstanding discourse about the need for research methodology in nursing that includes the whole, the researcher experience is often excluded in nursing research reporting.

Researchers have often questioned the adequacy of traditional research methods to answer practice questions important for the discipline of nursing (Leininger, 1985; Munhall & Oiler, 1986; Newman, 1979; Tinkle & Beaton, 1983). And in 1985, Tilden and Tilden proposed a philosophy of research in which, rather than the participant observation method of standing outside the research, the researcher becomes involved with the participant. The authors suggested that, "by conducting research while avoiding personal engagement, a person risks being merely a spectator of the human process, and thus risks producing trivial results" (p. 90).

Silva (1977) also questioned whether "scientific method too often sacrifices meaningfulness for rigor" (p. 63). She encouraged a holistic approach to research that included introspection and intuition. In a similar vein, DeGroot (1988) suggested that nursing practice issues require a model uninhibited by traditional research patterns. Her idea of a method that employed frank recognition of the individual researcher in the creative research process employed attention to personal experience, self-exploration, self-knowledge, and intuition.

More recently, discourse on method in nursing acknowledges the participation of the researcher. Schutz (1994) says, "The active and purposeful use of the researcher as an individual, not just as a tool to gather data but as an integral part of the field being studied, needs to be established in nursing research" (p. 415). Research methods that recognize the researcher are being advocated to a greater extent. Action research (Moch, Roth, Pederson, Groh-Demers, & Siler, 1994), praxis research (Connor, 1998; Lutz, Jones, & Kendall, 1997; Newman, 1990; Oiler Boyd, 1993) and combinations of methods such as oral reflective analysis (Thompson & Barrett, 1997) and increased reflexivity (Lamb & Huttlinger, 1989) have been discussed. Attention to the researcher as participant has also been promoted by Endo (1998), Litchfield (1993, 1997), Moch (1990a, 1990b), and Newman (1990, 1994, 1997).

Webb (1984), in describing the use of feminist methodology in nursing, discussed her process in conducting a study of the experience of hysterectomy. She discussed the difficulty of setting up and carrying out the study within the medical domination of the research environment. During the research, Webb struggled with the dilemmas when the women criticized their treatment. She realized through the study how important acknowledging the personal experience of the researcher is to the research.

Drew (1989) was one of the first researchers to acknowledge the researcher experience in nursing publications. Drew explained, "The disregard of experience is part of the natural standpoint in our culture . . . not much time is spent reflecting on the process of achieving an end" (p. 438). She described how her experience was data in her phenomenological research. Through data from research published earlier, in another report (Drew, 1986), Drew described how "the end result of any study is intimately connected with the process of investigation and the investigator's subjective experience of that study" (p. 438).

I acknowledged my own experience in the research process in my dissertation research (Moch, 1988) and to a limited extent in the published research report on the topic (Moch, 1990a). Through review of the researcher notes, tape recordings of responses to the interviews, and poetry written throughout the research, themes of knowing another, awe and respect for the other, and further knowing of oneself were identified. In a more recent publication of the same research, written as a book for the general public (Moch, 1995), I shared much more about the researcher experience.

The researcher experience of struggling with the relationship between researcher and informant has been identified by Wilde (1992). Through her research report on nurses' descriptions of difficult, challenging, and satisfying experiences at work, Wilde reflects on the researcher role. The research report, published in the *Journal of Advanced Nursing,* includes examples of the difficulty with being a so-called objective interviewer and provides ideas for resolving the role conflict. One such suggestion is:

> It is difficult and disadvantageous for the nurse researcher to maintain a detached relationship with the informant in qualitative research. Self-disclosure by the researcher has an enhancing effect on information exchange and results in a more honest and meaningful sharing by the informant. (Wilde, 1992, p. 240)

Rew, Bechtel, and Sapp (1993) propose self-as-instrument in qualitative research and through the proposal, suggest researcher characteristics important for the process. The authors suggest "The inherent value of human beings and their intersubjective experiences underscore the significance of the use of self-as-instrument in qualitative inquiry" (p. 301).

Recently, Gardner (1996) discussed the nurse researcher as an added dimension to research method. Using examples from research interviews, Gardner connects clinician, researcher, and interviewer roles in a manner that values the experience and knowledge of each. Through the discussion in *Nursing Inquiry,* Gardner proposes use of all three roles as important to the generation of knowledge related to the practice of nursing.

RESEARCH EXPERIENCE REPORTS
IN SOCIOLOGY JOURNALS

A gold mine for researcher experiences in journals is the journal, *Qualitative Sociology.* In the early 1980s, the journal published works that included the researcher experience and continues to do so today. Studies of a Midwestern lesbian community by Krieger (1985) and women's experiences with amniocentesis for prenatal diagnosis by Rothman (1986) led these researchers to examinations in interaction with the studied populations. Such examinations produced increased awareness of self intertwined with the group studied, as suggested by Krieger (1985):

In social science, I think, we must acknowledge the personal far more than we do. We need to find new ways to explore it. We need to link our statements about those we study with statements about ourselves, for in reality neither stands alone. (p. 321)

Arendell (1997), in a recent article titled "Reflections on the Researcher-Researched Relationship: A Woman Interviewing Men," discusses her own experience of interviewing men who were angry about recent divorces. Acknowledging that the researcher experience is rarely shared, Arendell described her feelings and uneasiness in situations with some men interviewed in her research.

Zola (1991) advocated the use of self in research in a provocative essay, titled "Bringing Our Bodies and Ourselves Back in: Reflections on a Past, Present and Future 'Medical Sociology,' " published in the *Journal of Health and Social Behavior*. Zola discusses the distancing and lack of self-disclosure evident in sociological research reports. He promotes a willingness to identify what the experience of research means to the researcher. He says, "Rather we must look at that experience—the anxieties, fears, delights, repulsions—as part of the very situation we are trying to understand " (p. 9).

In a discussion of his research, Davidman (1997) acknowledges his role through his research with his participants in an article in *Qualitative Sociology*. He says,

My interviews for this project provided a context in which I participated with my respondents in creating narratives that make sense of their disrupted biographies and tie together the diverse parts of their lives, while doing the same for myself. (p. 512)

RESEARCH EXPERIENCE AS REPORTED IN WOMEN'S STUDIES JOURNALS

Discussion about the researcher experience is frequent in women's studies journals. The discussion, however, is usually in reference to a feminist method or is included in an essay about the personal. For instance, a discussion of "Graduate Women on the Brink: Writing as 'Outsiders Within,' " includes reflection about the connections between the personal and social and intellectual issues (Aronson & Swanson, 1991). Another discussion was included in *Women's Studies Quarterly* through which authors acknowledge their own subjectivity in sharing their research (Alexander, Bunkers, & Muhanji, 1989).

RESEARCHER EXPERIENCES
IN *NARRATIVE STUDY OF LIVES*

An excellent collection of articles on the researcher experience is edited by Josselson (1996a) in the *Ethics and Process* volume of Narrative Study of Lives series. This new series of books provides a location for publishing aspects of the researcher experience and, in fact, encourages such in the author guidelines. The guidelines state that "discussion of the authors's place in the study" is welcome. In this volume, the editor invites "those who expose others' lives to expose themselves—the process of their work and their thoughts and feelings, their anxieties and concerns" in conducting research (Josselson, 1996a, p. xiii). In her self-analytic reflections, Josselson (1996b) says, "But I worry intensely about how people will feel about what I write about them" (p. 62). Josselson further exposes herself in telling about the guilt she feels when taking herself out of relationship with her participants and instead forms relationships with the readers. But, according to Josselson, shame is the hardest of her feelings. "I suspect this shame is about my exhibitionism, shame that I am using these people's lives to exhibit myself, my analytical prowess, my cleverness" (p. 70).

Chase (1996) discusses personal vulnerability as a narrative researcher. Despite an interest in maintaining relationship with the participants, Chase acknowledges the need for the author to assume interpretive authority in writing the research. Concerns about the experience and reactions of participants are voiced by Chase (1996), Josselson (1996b), and Miller (1996) in the same volume. In addition, Miller identifies dialogue to aid in the self-reflection and ethical questioning in narrative research. Recognizing the importance of dialogue with self, participant, and others and the mutuality of the research process is important, he states,

> Both researcher and participant are on a search—engaged in a project of exploration and inquiry. In this context, it might be said that together they form the unit of inquiry. Each is attempting to both discover the other and rediscover the self in the other in a mutual process of understanding and interpretation. (Miller, 1996, p. 138)

RESEARCH EXPERIENCE ESSAYS

Essays in book form by Krieger (1996) and Moustakas (1995) have been discussed earlier. Moustakas's book, *Being-In, Being-For, Being-With,* is a collection of essays about his efforts to include his experience in his research throughout his career. Other researcher experiences have been recorded in an edited book, *Encounter and Experience: Personal Accounts of Fieldwork,* by Beteille and Madan (1975). In the introductory essay, the authors discuss the importance of the subjective element in anthropology, such as the researcher's personality, education, and cultural background. The authors argue, "To seek to eliminate the supposedly distorting role of the observer's subjectivity, if at all possible, would destroy the most precious of our tools—the fieldworker himself" (p. 6).

Rose (1990), in *Living the Ethnographic Life,* describes how some authors have discussed the research experience in the preface of research reports in books. The research experience is expressed as a new view in reporting the research. The intent of the author is to demonstrate how the researchers suggested a new view for ethnographers. The new view is "a critique of the West, a reading that runs counter to the hegemonic, the colonial, or the oppressive" (p. 38). Personal accounts of how this new view came to them through their research are summarized by Rose.

Often, essays include discussion about the many roles played by the researcher in conducting research. For instance, Cartwright and Limandri (1997) discuss difficulties with the clinician and researcher role. They say, "The research relationship is an interactional process that merits examination for the effect it has on the nature of the data collected and the discoveries generated by the analysis" (p. 233).

RESEARCH EXPERIENCE AS POEMS

Years ago, Watson (1985) suggested that ways of conducting research in nursing must fit better with the holistic, caring perspective of nursing. Her idea that literary, poetry, and artistic works were more helpful in articulating knowledge in nursing has been implemented often in nursing since then. Many nursing researchers have used artistic means for expressing findings in nursing research (Munhall & Oiler Boyd, 1993; Nelson, 1996; Prediger, 1996). Watson (1985) demonstrated use of poetry to explain her research in her book, *Nursing: Human Science and Human Care.* She shared a poem she wrote through her research of the Wongi Tribe of Cundeelee, which she does not describe as her research report, but she says,

> In reflecting back on my field notes, the data and the entire experience, the poetic expression formulated on the overnight train ride captures the truth of the experience and the meaning of the human phenomena better than any of the factual data that are described without any feeling of personal involvement. (Watson, 1985, p. 93)

One of my poems, published as a letter to the editor (Moch, 1997), describes my reflections on reporting research findings. In it, I described how, through my research reporting, I was expected to use the rules of science, but how my work with the women describing their experiences with breast cancer was much more like art.

Qualitative Sociology published an argument about poetry "reports" for research. Schwalbe (1995) opposed the use of poetry in sociology, but a response by Denzin (1996) demonstrated how poetry was used in anthropology and further suggested that sociology remain open to new ways of expression in sociological writing through his essay titled, "Punishing Poets."

In this chapter, researcher experiences reported in books, journals, essays, and poetry have been described. Literature from several different disciplines, especially nursing, sociology, and women's studies, is included.

REFERENCES

Alexander, I., Bunkers, S., & Muhanji, C. (1989). A conversation on studying and writing about women's lives using nontraditional methodologies. *Women's Studies Quarterly, 17*, 99-114.

Arendell, T. (1997). Reflections on the researcher-researched relationship: A woman interviewing men. *Qualitative Sociology, 20*, 341-368.

Aronson, A. L., & Swanson, D. L. (1991, Fall/Winter). Graduate women on the brink: Writing as "outsiders within." *Women's Studies Quarterly, 19*, 156-173.

Behar, R. (1993). *Translated woman*. Boston: Beacon.

Behar, R. (1996). *The vulnerable observer: Anthropology that breaks your heart*. Boston: Beacon.

Bergum, V. (1989). Being a phenomenological researcher. In J. M. Morse (Ed.), *Qualitative nursing research: A contemporary dialogue* (pp. 43-57). Rockville, MD: Aspen.

Beteille, A., & Madan, T. N. (Eds.) (1975). *Encounter and experience: Personal accounts of fieldwork*. Delhi, India: Vikas.

Bowers, B. J. (1987). Intergenerational caregiving: Adult caregivers and their aging parents. *Advances in Nursing Science, 9*(2), 20-31.

Bowers, B. J. (1988). Grounded theory. In B. Sarter (Ed.), *Paths to knowledge: Innovative research methods for nursing* (pp. 33-59). New York: National League for Nursing.

Cartwright, J., & Limandri, B. (1997). The challenge of multiple roles in the qualitative clinician researcher-participant client relationship. *Qualitative Health Research, 7*(2), 223-235.

Chase, S. E. (1996). Personal vulnerability and interpretive authority in narrative research. In R. Josselson (Ed.), *Ethics and process in the narrative study of lives* (The Narrative Study of Lives, Vol. 4, pp. 45-59). Thousand Oaks, CA: Sage.

Connor, M. J. (1998). Expanding the dialogue on praxis in nursing research and practice. *Nursing Science Quarterly, 11*(2), 51-55.

Davidman, L. (1997). The personal, the sociological, and the intersection of the two. *Qualitative Sociology, 20*, 507-515.

DeGroot, H. A. (1988). Scientific inquiry in nursing: A model for a new age. *Advance in Nursing Science, 10*(3), 1-21.

Denzin, N. K. (1996). Punishing poets. *Qualitative Sociology, 19*(4), 525-528.

Drew, N. (1986). Exclusion and confirmation: A phenomenology of patients' experiences with caregivers. *Image: Journal of Nursing Scholarship, 18,* 39-43.

Drew, N. (1989). The interviewer's experience as data in phenomenological research. *Western Journal of Nursing Research, 11,* 431-439.

Endo, E. (1998). Pattern recognition as a nursing intervention with Japanese women with ovarian cancer. *Advances in Nursing Science, 20*(4), 49-61.

Gardner, G. (1996). The nurse researcher: An added dimension to qualitative research methodology. *Nursing Inquiry, 3,* 153-158.

Krieger, S. (1985). Beyond "subjectivity": The use of the self in social science. *Qualitative Sociology, 8*(4), 309-324.

Krieger, S. (1991). *Social science and the self.* New Brunswick, NJ: Rutgers University Press.

Krieger, S. (1996). *The family silver: Essays on relationships among women.* Berkeley: University of California Press.

Josselson, R. (Ed.). (1996a). Introduction. In R. Josselson (Ed.), *Ethics and process in the narrative study of lives* (The Narrative Study of Lives, Vol. 4, pp. xi-xviii). Thousand Oaks, CA: Sage.

Josselson, R. (Ed.). (1996b). On writing other people's lives. In R. Josselson (Ed.), *Ethics and process in the narrative study of lives* (The Narrative Study of Lives, Vol. 4, pp. 60-71). Thousand Oaks, CA: Sage.

Lamb, G. S., & Huttlinger, K. (1989). Reflexivity in nursing research. *Western Journal of Nursing Research, 11,* 765-772.

Leininger, M. M. (1985). *Qualitative research methods in nursing.* Orlando, FL: Grune & Stratton.

Litchfield, M. C. (1993). *The process of health patterning in families with young children who have been repeatedly hospitalized.* Unpublished master's thesis, University of Minnesota, Minneapolis.

Litchfield, M. C. (1997). *The process of nursing partnership in family health.* Unpublished doctoral dissertation, University of Minnesota, Minneapolis.

Lutz, K. F., Jones, K. D., & Kendall, J. (1997). Expanding the praxis debate: Contributions to clinical inquiry. *Advances in Nursing Science, 20*(2), 23-31.

Miller, M. E. (1996). Ethics and understanding through interrelationship. In R. Josselson (Ed.), *Ethics and process in the narrative study of lives* (The Narrative Study of Lives, Vol. 4, pp. 129-147). Thousand Oaks, CA: Sage.

Moch, S. D. (1988). *Health in illness: Experiences with breast cancer.* Unpublished doctoral dissertation, University of Minnesota, Minneapolis.

Moch, S. D. (1990a). Health within the experience of breast cancer. *Journal of Advanced Nursing, 15,* 1426-1435.

Moch, S. D. (1990b). Personal knowing: Evolving research and practice in nursing. *Scholarly Inquiry for Nursing Practice: An International Journal, 4,* 155-165.

Moch, S. D. (1995). *Breast cancer: Twenty women's stories.* New York: National League for Nursing Press.

Moch, S. D. (1997). Letter to the editor: Researcher as artist and scientist. *Journal of Holistic Nursing, 15*(3), 225-226.

Moch, S. D., Roth, D., Pederson, A., Groh-Demers, L., & Siler, J. (1994). Healthier work environments through action research. *Nursing Management, 25*(9), 38-40.

Moustakas, C. (1990). *Heuristic research: Design, methodology, and applications.* Newbury Park, CA: Sage.

Moustakas, C. (1995). *Being-in, being-for, being-with.* Northvale, NJ: Jason Aronson.

Munhall, P. L., & Oiler, C. (1986). *Nursing research: A qualitative perspective.* Norwalk, CT: Appleton-Century-Crofts.

Munhall, P. L. & Oiler Boyd, C. (1993). *Nursing research: A qualitative perspective* (2nd ed.). New York: National League for Nursing Press.

Nelson, J. P. (1996). Struggling to gain meaning: Living with the uncertainty of breast cancer. *Advances in Nursing Science, 18*(3), 59-76.

Newman, M. A. (1979). *Theory development in nursing.* Philadelphia: F. A. Davis.

Newman, M. A. (1990). Newman's theory of health as praxis. *Nursing Science Quarterly, 3*(1), 37-41.

Newman, M. A. (1994). *Health as expanding consciousness* (2nd ed.). New York: National League for Nursing Press.

Newman, M. A. (1997). Experiencing the whole. *Advances in Nursing Science, 20*(1), 34-39.

Oiler Boyd, C. (1993). Toward a nursing practice research method. *Advances in Nursing Science, 16*(2), 9-25.

Paterson, J. G., & Zderad, L. T. (1976). *Humanistic nursing.* New York: John Wiley.

Prediger E. (1996). Womanspirit: A journey into healing through art in breast cancer. *Advances in Nursing Science, 18*(3), 48-58.

Reinharz, S. (1979). *On becoming a social scientist.* San Francisco: Jossey-Bass.

Reinharz, S. (1992). *Feminist methods in social research,* New York: Oxford University Press.

Rew, L., Bechtel, D., & Sapp, A. (1993). Self-as-instrument in qualitative research. *Nursing Research, 42,* 300-301.

Rose, D. (1990). *Living the ethnographic life* (Qualitative Research Methods, vol. 23). Newbury Park, CA: Sage.

Rothman, B. K. (1986). Reflections: On hard work. *Qualitative Sociology, 9*(1), 48-53.

Schutz, S. E. (1994). Exploring the benefits of a subjective approach in qualitative nursing research. *Journal of Advanced Nursing, 20,* 412-417.

Schwalbe, M. (1995). The responsibilities of sociological poets. *Qualitative Sociology, 18,* 393-413.

Silva, M. C. (1977). Philosophy, science, theory: Interrelationships and implications for nursing research. *Image: Journal of Nursing Scholarship, 9*(3), 59-63.

Smith, C. D., & Kornblum, W. (1996). *In the field: Readings on the field research experience* (2nd ed.). Westport, CT: Praeger.

Thompson, S. M., & Barrett, P. A. (1997). Summary oral reflective analysis: A method for interview data analysis in feminist qualitative research. *Advances in Nursing Science, 20*(2), 55-65.

Tilden, V. P., & Tilden, S. (1985). The participant philosophy in nursing science. *Image: Journal of Nursing Scholarship, 17*(3), 88-90.

Tinkle, M. B., & Beaton, J. L. (1983). Toward a new view of science: Implications for nursing research. *Advances in Nursing Science, 5*(2), 27-36.

Watson, J. (1985). *Nursing: Human science and human care.* Norwalk, CT: Appleton-Century-Crofts.

Webb, C. (1984). Feminist methodology in nursing research. *Journal of Advanced Nursing, 9,* 249-256.

Wilde, V. (1992). Controversial hypotheses on the relationship between researcher and informant in qualitative research. *Journal of Advanced Nursing, 17,* 234-242.

Zola, I. K. (1991). Bringing our bodies and ourselves back in: Reflections on a past, present and future "medical sociology." *Journal of Health and Social Behavior, 32,* 1-16.

12

Suggestions for Reporting in Health Care Research

Susan Diemert Moch

Marie F. Gates

This chapter includes suggestions for reporting the research experience in health care research. Ideas for how to report the research experience are also included in other chapters in this book. For instance, in Chapter 13, Pierce integrates her experience in a description of the process of her research. Ochberg, in Chapter 10, identifies his thoughts throughout the analysis of his findings, and Gross, in Chapter 14, describes ways that she regularly integrates her personal experiences with her research through her writing.

Further ideas for reporting the research experiences, especially in health care, are discussed in this chapter. The ideas include Internet or list discussion groups, integrating the experience into various aspects of the research report, reporting the researcher experience in a separate section, and writing essays or poetry. Essays could be encouraged by having a section in the journal titled "Reflections on the Researcher Experience." Researchers could pool field notes regarding research on similar topics and analyze them for information on the researcher experience on specific topics. Letters to the editor requesting researcher experience information could be encouraged, and interviews with researchers, as demonstrated by Elsbach in Chapter 6, include other ideas. In addition to reporting through the mechanism of writing, reporting at professional conferences is discussed.

INTERNET OR LIST DISCUSSIONS

E-mail provides an easy way for researchers to dialogue about their researcher experience. Both authors of this book have enlisted other researchers for dialogue via computer. Moch made an agreement with another researcher to share researcher experiences on the research process as both were involved in similar research at the same time. The authors agreed to dialogue about their research via computer and communicated regularly about their own processing. The process of sharing was helpful to the researchers. And the researchers, Moch and Litchfield, have copies of their computer dialogue for possible analysis in the future.

Gates worked with a doctoral student in Memphis, Tennessee, who developed a resource guide for using the Internet to explore others' responses to ethical and other kinds of researcher experiences in conducting qualitative research (Fudge, 1994). Bunting, Russell, and Gregory (1998) reported on a project in which they synthesized the concept of protective caregiving via use of E-mail. This strategy could be used by researchers seeking resolution or processing of experiences related to conducting or analyzing qualitative research, as well.

List discussion groups provide a more formal, specific opportunity for dialoguing. Researchers can share their experiences with other researchers who volunteer for the same activity. The group can be available to the researcher when the researcher is available to discuss via computer. The researcher gains ideas from other researchers and can find support for the research endeavor.

INTEGRATING THE RESEARCHER EXPERIENCE WITH ASPECTS OF THE RESEARCH REPORT

Limited opportunities exist for the incorporation of researcher experience in the research report in journals (see Chapter 11). Where manuscript editors and reviewers are open to the inclusion of this experience, several possibilities exist for doing so.

Integration could occur throughout the manuscript. An introduction that includes a brief description of the researcher experience could initiate the article. The author could then acknowledge her or his own personal theoretical background in the framework section. As the methodology section is presented, the researcher could describe the ways in which the qualitative data were recorded and how the researcher was affected through data collection. In the analysis section, the researcher could acknowledge how the researcher could have affected the analysis. The findings section could incorporate questions and interpretations the researcher asked as interpretation occurred. Last, the discussion section is a most likely place for inclusion of any or all of the aforementioned areas.

REPORTING THE EXPERIENCE IN A SEPARATE SECTION

Including a separate section on the researcher experience may be the most effective way to increase reporting the researcher experience. By having a separate section, the researcher clearly acknowledges that the researcher experience is important to the research report. Suggested titles for this separate section might be "Researcher Experience," "Other Dimensions of the Research," or "Toward Integration of the Researcher Experience." In this separate section, the researcher would discuss the experience in whichever phase of the research the experience itself played the key role.

WRITING ESSAYS OR POETRY

Another way to report the experience is through essays and poetry. We suspect that many researchers write essays or personal or research journal entries about the researcher experience but rarely discuss them with others. Essays like some of the chapters in this book should be encouraged, not only for teaching novice researchers but also for presenting an important aspect of research. Without knowing more about the research experience, an important perspective, valuable to the findings of the research, is lost.

Tales about doing research are essential for teaching qualitative research. Professors often share intimate stories about their research with students in teaching the research process. However, the stories are rarely reported further than the classroom. These stories may be important for understanding the whole of the research. Sometimes, research textbooks and edited books on the research process include information about the research experience (see Chapter 11). These stories could also be published in journals for greater access to research colleagues.

Qualitative research journals could include a regular section for publishing essays or experiences with research. Currently, some journals have sections on methodology, ethics, or book reviews. Having a section titled, "Reflections on the Researcher Experience" could uncover helpful knowledge that others could use as they conduct their research. Such a section could encourage researchers to consider their experiences important for publication. Soliciting essays for such a section by a journal editor would encourage greater inclusion in the reporting of the research itself.

Poetry provides an important venue for expressing the researcher experience. Many researchers, however, do not use the medium for expression, and most research journals do not publish poetry. Moch often writes poetry to express experiences with clients through her research or to express the whole of her research experience. She has tried to get her poetry published in research or practice-related journals. One such journal published a poem as a letter to the editor (Moch, 1997).

SYNTHESIS OF FIELD NOTES

Another possibility for inclusion of the researcher experience is through a synthesis of field notes on the same research topic. Researchers working on a similar topic could share field notes or field journals about the research experience. A synthesis of these field notes could provide important knowledge. Data from several research studies are often combined to elicit patterns occurring across studies. A synthesis of "data" in field notes could also assist in identifying patterns of researcher experiences which could contribute the knowledge on a specific topic.

LETTERS TO THE EDITOR

Letters to the editor encouraging questions to the researcher about the researcher experience could be included in journals. For example, if a researcher conducts studies on the experience of breast cancer survivorship and an article by another researcher focusing on the same area is published, the researcher could write a letter to the editor requesting information from the author about the researcher experience. An important exchange for the area of study may emerge through such a format.

RESEARCHER INTERVIEWS

In Chapter 6, Elsbach demonstrated how learning takes place by reading about the experiences of other researchers. Experienced researchers could be interviewed about their research experience and then summaries could be published in journals. Some experienced researchers write books of essays on their career experience with research and provide information on their experience with research (See Chapter 11). However, these collections of essays are not generally as accessible as reports in journals. Also, writing essay books does not lend as much credibility to the researcher experience as published interviews in research journals.

OPPORTUNITIES FOR REPORTING EXPERIENCES AT CONFERENCES

Mechanisms currently exist to foster knowledge and understanding among novice qualitative researchers at discipline-specific research conferences. Methodology seminars or meetings with experienced mentors in the field are often features of such conferences. It would be helpful to extend those kinds of opportunities to understanding the processing of the researcher experience, as well. The international qualitative research conferences, with the opportunities for interdisciplinary discussions, would be especially useful places for such seminars or meetings to occur. Soliciting papers for extended discussion on the researcher experience by a panel of experienced researchers could be a valuable addition to such conferences.

CONCLUSION

When we, the coauthors of this book, presented preliminary discussion of the proposed topic for this book at a poster session at a qualitative conference (Moch & Gates, 1998), students from psychology, sociology, nursing, management, and medicine stopped by to discuss their wish for more opportunities to explore the possibilities inherent in discussion of the researcher experience. Our hope for this book is to encourage discussion and reflection about the researcher experience. Even though the focus of this chapter has been on health care research, some of these suggestions may apply to other disciplines. Through discussion of the ideas presented, we hope to generate more ideas for reporting the researcher experience in health care and in other areas.

REFERENCES

Bunting, S. M., Russell, C. K., & Gregory, D. M. (1998). Use of electronic mail (E-mail) for concept synthesis: An international collaborative project. *Qualitative Health Research, 8,* 128-135.

Fudge, P. (1994). *Internet culture and ethics: Navigating the Internet.* Unpublished manual, University of Tennessee, Memphis.

Moch, S. D. (1997). Letter to the editor: Researcher as artist and scientist. *Journal of Holistic Nursing, 15,* 225-236.

Moch, S. D., & Gates, M. F. (1998, February). *Reporting the reseacher experience.* Poster session presented at the Qualitative Health Research Conference, Edmonton, Canada.

13

Lawyers, Lethal Weapons, and Ethnographic Authority

Reflections on Fieldwork for *Gender Trials*

Jennifer L. Pierce

I think one of my greatest anxieties I faced as a novice ethnographer was about "getting it right." I worried about the stories people told me and whether I had captured them accurately, fairly, judiciously, etc., etc. "Did I get it right? Did I get it right," I constantly asked myself. And, I tried so hard to write down absolutely everything. . . . What I began to realize as time went on was that if I wasn't getting it right, some folks had ways of making sure *that I did get it the way* they wanted me to get it.

Pierce lecture notes, 1997;
emphasis in the original.

Contemporary critical writing on ethnographic authority, particularly in anthropology, begins with the premise that ethnographers inescapably exercise textual and social authority over the people they study, particularly people who occupy

AUTHOR'S NOTE: An earlier version of this chapter appeared in the Sage anthology, *Studying Elites Using Qualitative Methods* (Hertz & Imber, 1995). Special thanks to Lisa Bower, Lisa Disch, Martha Easton, and Barbara Laslett for their critical comments on earlier drafts of this essay. The revised version has benefited from Sarah Elwood's suggestions.

subordinate social positions (Abu-Lughod, 1993; Behar, 1993, 1995; Clifford, 1988; Kondo, 1990). Anthropologist James Clifford (1988), for example, suggests that ethnographic texts produce subjectivities in an unequal exchange between anthropologists and "natives." Within this asymmetrical relationship, ethnographers typically provide the final, authoritative account. Some sociologists have also acknowledged the inequality in the relationship between the researcher and his or her subjects. Sociologists receive grants for research and write publications that further legitimate professional status, whereas the people they study often receive little in return for their participation (Blauner & Wellman, 1973, p. 316). Furthermore, as feminist scholar Sue Wise (1987) has argued, "We are still operating in an environment where the ethic prevails that those who publish research are the experts and those who are written about are not" (p. 76).

Attentive to these issues, recent feminist discussions of ethnographic practice have explored fieldwork and rhetorical strategies that attempt to disrupt these asymmetrical power relations (Abu-Lughod, 1993; Kondo, 1990; Minh-Ha, 1989; Stacey, 1988, 1990). For example, in her book *Brave New Families*, Judith Stacey described her attempts to involve the white, working-class women she studied in reading and commenting on her book-length manuscript about their lives. Though these women had criticisms of the text, they concede that the book is hers—not theirs—thus relinquishing authority to Stacey's voice. In response, Stacey despairs a fully feminist ethnography.[1]

Like Stacey (1988, 1990), I doubt that any research relationship could be truly egalitarian. However, in contrast to the researcher positioning script depicted by Stacey, Clifford (1988), and others, I argue that asymmetrical relations between researcher and his or her "objects" of study are not always so clear-cut. In my own fieldwork, my positioning within this formulation sometimes fit the researcher-dominant, subject-subordinate script, but at others, it did not. As a generic ethnographer, I exercised textual authority over those I studied. On the other hand, as a female ethnographer conducting research on male litigators, I "studied up." Not only did I study an elite and powerful group of professionals, but my research focused on people who occupy the dominant gender position. As a woman studying men in a predominantly male profession,[2] sexist expectations and jokes, sexual innuendoes, and occasional outbursts of hostility served as constant reminders of my subordinate status. How does ethnographic authority play out in a field setting where the relations of power and authority between researcher and subjects are more complex?

In this chapter, I argue that the classic conception of ethnographic authority obscures the varied ways the researcher's power and authority can shift and change in differing relationships and situations in the field. As an ethnographer, I often had the power to define the reality of others, but as a woman, this authority was often challenged and (re)negotiated in interactions with the male elites I studied. I reflect on this contested process by drawing from my fieldwork experiences in two San Francisco law firms, where I spent over 15 months working as a paralegal in 1988 and 1989 for my book, *Gender Trials: Emotional Lives in Contemporary Law Firms* (Pierce, 1995). At the time, legal workers in both firms knew that I was conducting interviews for a dissertation on occupational stress; however, they did not know that I was *also* doing fieldwork. My covert status as a fieldworker not only raised serious ethical questions,[3] but it also brought to light a tension between my feelings about exploiting the people—especially the very powerful people—I studied and my commitment to doing ethnographic research.

In the following, I explore these issues, beginning with a discussion of my feelings about the unacknowledged exploitation of my research subjects. My early fieldwork experiences were marked by a pervasive feeling of guilt and anxiety about the potential betrayal of my subjects. However, as time went on, these feelings shifted from guilt to resentment and anger. Here, anger served as an epiphanal moment[4] in shifting my thinking about the nature of ethnographic authority. The tension between my subordinate gender positioning in the field and my authorial voice as a feminist sociologist strained and shifted, and my authorial voice emerged as a "lethal weapon." The next section details a new move in my shifting positions in the field. Here, my ethnographic authority is acknowledged, and I develop a new term for this position: the "outlaw." The outlaw position is a multiple and discontinuous identity whose movement between positions proves to be a critical advantage in uncovering the regimes of power[5] in the workplace. Furthermore, I suggest that it is *through the responses I elicit in my movement between positions*—from female paralegal to outlaw—that I unveil the complex operations of gender and power in the field. Last, I discuss how issues of inequality and exploitation become more complex when ethnographic authority does not follow the usual script. When women study men, what is a lethal weapon for some can be a potent methodological tool for researchers.

My feelings about the potential exploitation of my subjects varied over the length of my duration in the field. Ironically, the longer I was in the field and the more I became involved in people's lives, the less I worried about this issue. By contrast, at the beginning, I was acutely sensitive to the asymmetry in my relations with others. It was clear to me what I would get out of the research—a dissertation to fulfill my PhD requirements and, eventually, a book—but what would they get out of it? Every early personal confidence drove me wild with anxiety. People readily confided their personal troubles to me. What was I to do with such personal information? Was I betraying them, even as I promised confidentiality?

The following excerpt from my field notes highlights the guilt and anxiety I experienced when one of my subjects revealed personal feelings about his work.

Early in the field, during a long car drive to an interview with a potential trial witness, Stan,[6] one of the lawyers I worked for, confided his fears about turning 40 and his personal assessments about what he had accomplished in his career. In my notes, I recorded the following:

> After reviewing the background of the witness and discussing the possible testimony we might uncover to bolster our case, our conversation took a more personal turn. Stan asked me what I would like to do if I wasn't in graduate school. . . . I thought for a minute and said, "A rock 'n roll star." I explained it was a pretty farfetched fantasy given that I am practically tone deaf, but I love to sing anyway. Then I returned the question. This opened a long discussion about his frustrations about being an attorney, how much work it was, and how little the psychological payoff is. "You do a great job, and no one cares. The client doesn't understand the intricacies of law well enough to know how well you've done. And, other lawyers bite the bullet in envy." At one point, he said his wife had told him that he shouldn't feel he has to prove himself so much to people, that he should learn to like himself as he is. He added that it was a "sweet thought," but that's not how law works. "In the real world, you have to keep on proving yourself if you want to stay on top." Thinking of the academic world, I felt inclined to agree, but I also sensed some truth in what his wife said. His constant need to prove himself didn't appear to result simply from some external pressure, but an inner insecurity which compelled him to prove himself again and again. I nodded assent, but said nothing. We drove the last 10 minutes of the trip in silence.
>
> Initially, I felt pleased that he had confided in me, but now, as I write this, I feel guilty. This was a highly personal revelation for someone who is typically emotionally closed and distant. He does not strike me as the type of person who makes such personal disclosures easily. On the other hand, why did he tell me? Am I just the sympathetic female ear? Or was he just in a funk, and I just happened to be the closest available body? (field notes)

Although the conversation had given me insight into the pressures trial lawyers face, I continued to feel somewhat uncomfortable after such disclosures were made. People trusted me, yet I felt that my note taking somehow betrayed that trust. This was further exacerbated by that fact that although most people knew I was doing a dissertation on occupational stress and the legal profession, they did not know that I was also doing participant observation. At least in interviews, the power relationship was somewhat apparent, but in fieldwork, it went unacknowledged.

Though early in my fieldwork I was acutely aware of my unacknowledged ethnographic authority, the longer I worked in the field, the less angst I experienced about this issue. The shift from guilt and anxiety to frustration, resentment, and anger came about for several reasons. First, I entered the field as a novice. My expectations about fieldwork were idealistic and naive. The formulaic guides I had read on participant observation had not prepared me for the moment-to-moment ethical dilemmas that arose in the field.[7] Second, as a novice, I also experienced confidences as personal. I assumed that people confided in me as another person—as an equal. In retrospect, I can also see that I responded to their problems and concerns as a traditional caretaking female. As a woman, I somehow felt responsible for taking care of their feelings.

What I began to realize over time is that male attorneys did not confide in me as a person but rather as a position in an imagined relation—as a feminized Other (de Beauvoir, 1949). In de Beauvoir's formulation, women are expected to tend to the needs of men, becoming Other or "object" to his Self or "subject." As de Beauvoir suggests, this positioning is not reciprocal but asymmetrical, because women's subjectivity is denied. Here, my early suspicions about being "the female sympathetic ear" were on the mark. Male attorneys talked about their problems, I listened. As these realizations dawned on me, I began to feel less guilty and more resentful of their expectations. Anger often served as the epiphanal moment in this realization.

In *Reflections on Fieldwork in Morocco*, anthropologist Paul Rabinow (1977) also describes how anger triggered a crucial moment in his field research and in his thinking about the role of the ethnographer. After a long day with his key informant, a Moroccan male, Rabinow lost his temper and yelled at the man. Initially, he was concerned that it may have damaged the relationship. However, as it turned out, the opposite occurred. Rabinow's initial passive, so-called scientific stance had been interpreted by his informant as a sign of weakness. Rabinow's subsequent angry outburst redefined his identity as a man of good character who would not submit to another man's efforts to dominate (pp. 47-48). As a white female ethnographer in U.S. society among largely white, male, middle-class lawyers, becoming angry did not have the same effect it did for the male anthropologist in Morocco. As the following examples illustrate, my slip into the "black hole" did not improve the quality of my relations with attorneys, though it did yield some insights about myself, the nature of ethnography, and the regimes of power governing work relations between female paralegals and male attorneys.

Todd, a young male associate, had the habit of hanging around in the office I shared with Pamela, another woman paralegal. He appeared to want and need attention. Whereas Pamela lavished him with attention, I found his personality and behavior childish and irritating and typically ignored him. One day when Pamela was at the courthouse, Todd sauntered into the office. We exchanged greetings, and then I asked him what he needed. "Oh nothing, I just came in to hang out," he responded with a broad smile. I said pointedly that I was working and returned to the stack of depositions sitting on my desk. He remained seated on Pamela's desk. I continued to do my work. After a moment or two of silence, he said, "You don't like me, do you, Jennifer?"

I looked up briefly and said with some heat, "That's right Todd, I don't like you." I heard him kind of laugh-gasp. Then he said, "Well, I'm completely crushed. That wasn't the response I was expecting at all." I looked up and smiled and laughed. Then I saw his face. He had this look of genuine surprise, and he was blushing. He quickly exited. (field notes)

As I described the incident later in my field notes, I began to feel guilty. I knew Todd was not a particularly malicious person, he was just insecure and wanted my attention. On the other hand, I had grown tired of his pointless interruptions. Personally, I did not like him, and I wanted to be left alone. Furthermore, I resented the assumption that I, as a woman paralegal, should be interested in devoting personal attention to him. Whereas this conversation did not improve my relations with Todd, at least from his perspective, it did from mine. Thenceforth, he left me alone, and I was able to complete my work without interruption. In addition, the incident helped me to understand the importance emotional norms play for the work lives of women paralegals. Todd clearly expected me, as a female paralegal, to pay attention to him. When I did not, he asked a question to remind me of my appropriate role—"You don't like me, do you, Jennifer?"—a question that suggested I had behaved inappropriately and at the same time invited reassurance. In other words, he not only expected me to apologize for not being friendlier to his overtures but to tell him that I liked him. In this light, my response can be read as a disruption of social norms. By refusing to play the role of the feminized Other, I subverted the informal norm for female paralegal behavior.

The reaction my anger elicited also underscores the differences between Rabinow's (1977) fieldwork experience and my own. For Rabinow, an angry outburst served to consolidate his masculinity, marking him as a man of strong character who refused to let another take advantage of him. It also helped to build, rather than damage, rapport with his informant. By contrast, my anger challenged Todd's traditional conceptions of femininity. My refusal to accept his understanding of appropriate feminine behavior not only served to unsettle, rather than consolidate, my "femininity," but it also created distance in our relationship. My confrontation with such sexist expectations marks the distinctiveness between my fieldwork experience and that of the male anthropologist. By virtue of being female, I was compelled to contend with attitudes and behavior that Rabinow was not. Our divergent gender positionings not only gave rise to differential experiences, but also explained why our common reaction—anger—was perceived in different ways. Anger is acceptable behavior for men but not for women.

A similar epiphany of anger occurred on a long workday with another male lawyer. On a particularly grueling day, the attorney I worked for had to file 10 *motions in limine* by 5 p.m. Our "team"—three paralegals, two associates, and two secretaries—began the day at 6 a.m. Some of the motions had been written the previous day, but six remained to be completed. I had serious doubts that our team would be able to finish them. But by 4:30 in the afternoon, all but one of the motions were printed out and ready to go. The remaining motion was still being revised by Daniel, the partner working on the case. Another paralegal and I sat waiting nervously for the pleading. At about 4:50, Daniel came running into the room, threw the motion at us, and screamed as we ran out the door to catch a cab to the courthouse: "And don't fuck up!"

The cabby drove us through rush hour traffic from the financial district to the courthouse. As we ran down the long hallway to the county clerk's office, the clock chimed 5 o'clock, and the office doors closed. I banged on the door, and we pleaded—more "emotional labor"[8]— with the clerk to let us file the motions even though we were technically 5 minutes late. The clerk finally relented, but only after chastising us severely. The other paralegal was so angry, he decided not to return to the office. I rode the cab back alone.

When I got back to the office, I went into Mark's office (one of the associates on our team) and laid on the floor—my back was killing me—and relayed the story. I was very tired and still very angry. He went off to get me something to drink. He returned with Daniel who asked pleasantly how things had gone. I said icily, "We didn't fuck up." He looked surprised, but said nothing and left. Mark laughed and told me that I'd probably get into trouble for a comment like that.

> Mark was right. The next day at our "team meeting," Daniel brought in gag gifts for all of us because we had done such a "great job." The associate [Mark] who smoked [but was trying to quit] received a torch-shaped cigarette lighter, the other paralegal got a miniature basketball hoop with a foam rubber basketball, and I received a plastic gun which shot bright orange ping pong balls, called "The Big Ball Blaster." Everyone, including Daniel, thought this was very funny. Although it was done as a joke, the joke was at my expense, and the message was clear— women paralegals who aren't nice are "ball blasters." (field notes)

Again, my icy retort did not improve my relationship with the attorney. However, my behavior did reveal informal norms about gender-appropriate emotional labor for paralegals. By telling the attorney that we didn't fuck up, I once again resisted the appropriate feminized position. I did not play the role of the supportive and good female paralegal but rather that of a ball blaster. Daniel, consciously or not, appeared to recognize my attempt to disrupt power relations. The gag gifts he presented to us, an unusual display of so-called gratitude on his part, reveal in a somewhat disguised form his actual intentions. First, because the gifts are gags, they are not genuine demonstrations of gratitude or appreciation but jokes. The joke served to reframe the moment as "humor," setting it apart from our ongoing, more serious work lives. And, as Freud (1963) suggested, jokes often contain an element of aggression. Presenting me with a toy gun and Mark, who is trying to quit smoking, with a large cigarette lighter are hardly gracious gestures but aggressive moves. Daniel's anger with me for talking back to him and with Mark for witnessing his loss of face was returned to us symbolically in the form of gag gifts. Second, as anthropologist Marcel Mauss (1954) suggests, by giving us gifts, Daniel attempts to reinstall his authority.

The meaning of my gift adds another twist to Mauss's (1954) analysis. *Ball blaster* is a pejorative term for a woman who acts like a man, or more accurately, a woman who castrates men and hence disempowers them. By giving me the gift, Daniel both reclaimed his authority and conferred abject status on me, signaling the inappropriateness of my behavior. Furthermore, as Mauss suggests, gift giving is a means of cementing social relationships. To refuse the gift would demonstrate not only ingratitude but withdrawal from social intercourse. In that moment, as a member of the team, I could not refuse. The possibility of my withdrawal was also forestalled by the frame of the joke—If I did not accept the gift and laugh at the joke, I become the ball-blasting bitch. And yet to laugh along and "to accept without returning or repaying more is to face subordination" (Mauss, 1954, p. 63).

Though I accepted the gift, I did not accept subordination. Here, power relations shifted again, and my authorial voice returned from the void of the repressed. I marched straight back to my office and attached the cardboard ball-blaster box top to my office door beneath my name plate—an attempt, in Judith Butler's (1993) terms, to reappropriate the intended slam and claim a new and affirmative meaning.[9] After all, ball blasters are powerful women. One of the paralegals who admired my new name plate added her own graffiti to the cardboard box top. Beneath the giant letters "BIG BALL BLASTER," it read, in tiny print, "shoots safe ping pong balls." She crossed this out with a big black X and wrote above it in ominous black letters: LETHAL WEAPON.

In recent writing in queer theory and critical race theory, there has been a move to (re)conceptualize the term *outlaw.* Kate Bornstein (1994), for example, uses the concept of *gender outlaw* to define "transgressively gendered" people. In reference to this term, Bornstein, a transsexual lesbian, describes herself in this way:

> I know that I'm not a man—about that much I'm very clear, and I've come to the conclusion that I'm probably not a woman either, at least not according to lot of people's rules on this sort of thing. (p. 4)

As a result of her borderline life as a transsexual, Bornstein has found that her identity has become more fluid, and her own need to be male, female, gay, or straight has become both less demanding and "more playful." In another context, critical race theorist Regina Austin (1989) uses the concept of the *black outlaw* to describe multiple and discontinuous identities that serve to destabilize the way legal doctrines attempt to establish firm racial classifications.

What I find useful about these conceptions is not only the notion that the outlaw is transgressive but that identity of the outlaw is multiple, fluid, and sometimes discontinuous. Methodologically, the critical advantage of this multiple subject or outlaw position lies in its creative and strategic movement in and around roles. In my own research, this meant moving in and around the roles of researcher, paralegal, feminist, and ball blaster. As the following examples from my fieldwork illustrate, although this movement may not always have been intentional or particularly playful, it did facilitate my attempt to unmask the deployment of power in the field.

Toward the end of my stint at the first field site, I ran into a situation where one of the attorneys clearly recognized that my critical and sociological understanding of working relations in the law firm was inconsistent with his own. At some point, this particular attorney, Michael, expressed interest in my dissertation prospectus. I naively assumed that he might find it interesting and provided a copy for him. As I discovered, he was highly offended by my literature review. Here is a synopsis of events from my field notes:

> He was really hurt because my prospectus, in his words, "portrays all these wonderful secretaries and paralegals who support these asshole attorneys." And how did I think he would respond, but to take it personally because (he raises his voice) "wasn't this really about me and Jane [his secretary] and Debbie [a paralegal]?" He added sneeringly, "And, it's so well-written and polished. All these footnotes and references. You must have spent a lot of time working on this." I said that I was sorry that I had hurt his feelings, but that had not been my intention at all. I tried to explain that I was interested in how the structure of the legal profession necessitated certain kinds of behavior, and I was interested in what the consequences were for people who were involved in such occupations. I further explained that all interviews would be confidential, as were the names of those interviewed and the law firms where they worked.
>
> He continued to say how much I had hurt his feelings. . . . Then he started talking about what a good interviewer I was. It's a "special skill." "Stan [attorney] calls six people and no one tells him anything. You call one person and we get everything we need to know." He went on to say that it was a valuable, but *dangerous* skill because people feel so comfortable talking to me that they might reveal a confidence they would later regret. (I think he was talking about himself here.) I told him that yes, I am a good interviewer and people do enjoy talking to me, but my dissertation interviews are confidential. And to top it off, as I am leaving, he tells me to never discuss our conversation with my thesis adviser. (Is this a sign of his guilt or embarrassment?)
>
> Over the weekend, I brooded about Michael's behavior. Although I had an inkling of why he was upset —he didn't like being an object of study—I couldn't figure out how a fairly straightforward literature review had produced this reaction.

Moreover, I felt he had been downright mean—the sneer about "it's so well-written" suggested that he had not perceived me as a skilled and competent researcher before he read the prospectus. Furthermore, his orders about what I could or could not say to my thesis adviser struck me as extremely controlling. His response strongly resembled adversarial tactics—the intimidation, the attempt to control and direct the witness (me). The more I thought about it, the more angry I became. After talking to my thesis adviser and a number of other people, I decided that it was time to leave the field site and find a new one. I had already accumulated voluminous field notes and completed the majority of my interviews. At the end of the weekend, I talked to the paralegal coordinator and told her I would finish the projects I had begun, but I was planning to quit.

[On Monday] when I came into the office, Michael did his best charm routine, lots of big smiles, "how are you's" and so on. When everyone else left the meeting, he said he had heard that I was angry with him. I said, "That's right." He said he'd like to talk to me about it later in the day. . . .

When I met with Michael, he said he wanted to clear the air. He was sorry if he had offended me and hoped we could be friendly. He repeated several time that he really liked me—*as if that were the issue.* "You are such a good paralegal." How could my feelings be hurt, he had said such glowing things about my research skills. I explained why [his insinuation that I wasn't smart was insulting and ordering me around. . .]. Rather than apologize again, he said, "Well, attorneys have feelings, too." He tried to conclude on an upbeat note, saying he was willing to put this behind us, they really need me for the upcoming trial, and everyone knows how much work I did interviewing all those witnesses. [I interviewed almost 40 witnesses in a 3-month period.]

I said that if I stayed, I would be very friendly and professional. I had no problems with that. However, I thought he should know that he was currently on my shit list. And [I added] people who are on my shit list have to do *lots* of penance to get off. He laughed in an overly hearty voice. (field notes; emphasis in original throughout)

This encounter highlights both the lawyer's recognition of my authority and my disruption of norms. By problematizing what he took for granted as natural, the work relationships and the nature of work in the law firm, I had hurt his feelings, made him feel angry, and betrayed his trust. My critical view also violated my subordinate status as a woman paralegal. Women legal assistants were supposed to be nice and supportive of attorneys. My prospectus and my role as researcher demonstrated that I was critical, detached, and even instrumental in disrupting the status quo. Not surprisingly, the attorney perceived this point of view as threatening. Michael's anger at me, however, gave way to a new step in this dance of shifting power and authority. After berating me on Friday, on Monday, his strategy was to call me in to talk to me and to smooth things over. He apologized for offending me and hoped we could be friendly. He complimented my work and appealed to me personally—he really liked me. Beneath the carefully scripted lines—his charm routine—was not only an effort to win me back—after all, they needed me for the trial—but an attempt to reinstate the status quo. By courting me back into the fold, he attempted to put me back in my proper place, the position of female paralegal.

I did not return to my proper place, however. Here, as in the ball-blaster story, I resisted his attempts to maneuver me there. Though I told Michael that I would continue to be friendly and professional, I also put him on notice by telling him that he was currently on my shit list. In this way, I disrupted the status quo he was attempting to reinstate and reasserted my authorial voice—this time, verbally. After all, what could be a more graphic representation of my ethnographic authority than telling him that I would write him in on my shit list with a "pocket signifier" (as some French feminists call the pen)? In reclaiming the pen, I reclaimed, as French feminist Helene Cixous (1981) suggests, the phallus. My bid for the phallus was further cemented by putting his behavior on notice—he had to do *lots* of penance to get off. Such a move not only displaces his authority but serves to position me as the final arbiter of appropriate behavior.

Whereas some lawyers viewed my research as threatening, secretaries and paralegals had an entirely different reaction. When I casually mentioned my dissertation topic, many eagerly volunteered to be interviewed. One woman accosted me in the bathroom, providing a list of reasons for why I should interview her. Others completely rejected the notion of confidentiality. As one secretary said repeatedly, "Use my real name. I want you to use my real name in your book." (Their bid for visibility in my text posed a stark contrast to the lawyers, many of whom refused to be tape recorded in their interviews and worried excessively about confidentiality.) These women legal workers also expressed curiosity in my written work. Much later, after an interview with one paralegal, she asked to see my prospectus and literature review. I was reluctant and explained why. However, because I had already done the interview and no longer worked in the firm where she did, I eventually relented and gave her a copy. She called me a week later and said, "No offense, Jennifer, but this thing is boring. How did Michael ever get riled up over this damn thing?"

The difference between the paralegal's response and Michael's is suggestive of their own positioning within regimes of power, as well as my own. Paralegals and lawyers occupy differential locations in the law firm hierarchy. And paralegals, unlike lawyers, saw my critical view as compatible with their own view from below. Many of the women I interviewed attempted to disrupt the status quo through their own strategies of resistance. It was another paralegal who penned "lethal weapon" on my nameplate.[10] Furthermore, these differing perceptions are also related to my positioning in the script on ethnographic authority. In relation to male attorneys, I was studying up from the subordinate gender position. At the same time, as the author, I penned the story. My efforts to write a story contradicting their stance is, not surprisingly, read as threatening or offensive or both.

The transgressive moves I made in my fieldwork and have described thus far are not intended simply to be provocative stories but rather, as Martha Easton (1994) suggests, as "a way to explore and explode the discursive structuring of expected gender behavior" (p. 20). By disrupting norms—unwittingly or not—I uncovered regimes of power governing gendered working relations in these law firms. Furthermore, as Easton suggests "special knowledges" are to be gained when it is women, and not men, who do research on men.

> When men hold the researcher position . . . the constructions of power behind masculinity are conflated with and obscured by the positional power of the researcher. However when women hold the researcher position, there is a strange inversion of and disruption of power by the researcher. (p. 22)[11]

In my own work, the strange inversion and disruption of power played out in the tension between my subordinate gender position and my authoritative researcher position. Given this positioning, my identities were both multiple— female-paralegal-researcher-ball blaster-feminist—and, at times, discontinuous—female paralegal doing research who was not seen as a researcher. For instance, even though Michael knew that I was doing research for my dissertation, it was not until he actually read my prospectus that he saw me as anything other than a female paralegal. The critical advantage of this multiple subject or outlaw position lies in its creative and strategic movement in and around the roles of researcher, paralegal, feminist, and ball blaster. Furthermore, *it is through the reactions I elicited* in my movement between positions—from female paralegal to outlaw—*that I unsettled the boundaries between gender and power.* Michael's reaction to my prospectus not only revealed for him a new way of seeing me—my ethnographic authority is unveiled—but it also laid bare his expectations about appropriate behavior for female paralegals. His surprise at my expertise and skill as a sociologist suggested that these skills were incommensurate with his expectations of the typical female paralegal role.

Some mainstream sociologists may object to my outlaw position in doing ethnography.[12] Indeed, the outlaw not only breaks the rules in the field but also the rules of a positivistic social science—detachment, neutrality, and objectivity.[13] Ethnographers who become overly involved with the people they study are considered not only disruptive but biased, partisan, and potentially contaminative influences in the field. However, to paraphrase Sherryl Kleinman and Martha Copp (1994), the crucial question in qualitative research is not, *Did* the researcher influence the study, but *How* did the researcher influence the study? My tales of the field not only articulated many of the ways my presence influenced the people I studied, but they also yielded important insights about gender, power, and knowledge. Through male lawyers' reactions to my outlaw position, I uncovered the operations of power and privilege that are never formally stated.[14] Todd's response to my unfriendliness, for example, was to ask me a question reminding me of my appropriate role—"You don't like me, do you, Jennifer?"—a question both suggesting that I behaved inappropriately and inviting reassurance. My reaction— "No, I don't like you"—in turn produced yet another step in this dance—"That wasn't the response I was expecting at all"— thus bringing the norm I have broken into bold relief. Similarly, Daniel's gag gift, his response to my talking back, revealed both his attempt to name my behavior as inappropriate and to reinstall the status quo.

Still others may object that the outlaw position is somehow sneaky, immoral, or unethical. Certainly, I do not always treat attorneys with great reverence or respect. And my behavior, as well as what I had written, did embarrass and offend some lawyers. But here again, we have to think critically about my gender position in relation to those I studied. European American social scientists, for instance, have been criticized for their exploitative research on communities of color. But what if the tables are turned—what if African Americans studied white communities? And what if women studied men? In a society strongly stratified by race and gender, the tables cannot be turned with an equivalent force. White women as well as women and men of color—even as researchers— are embedded within raced and gendered matrices of domination and privilege that have consequences for the responses their multiple subject positions—researcher, female, person of color, or a combination of these—provoke. In contrast to the experiences of white male researchers, these researchers are likely to encounter racism and sexism. Such incidences are far from respectful. And yet at the same time, these incidences also serve to reveal the complex and shifting operations of power in the field, thereby providing important clues in cracking the code of power and domination.

Last, the outlaw position challenges both new ethnographers and feminist scholars who despair the achievement of egalitarian research fieldwork methods. They are correct in arguing that the dilemma of ethnographic authority is unavoidable. However, this dilemma and its particular regime of power— researcher-dominant, subject-subordinate—must be considered in relation to other matrices of domination that may intersect with them, matrices shaped by race and gender relations. When the dilemma of ethnographic authority is an inversion, as Easton (1994) suggests, concerns about inequality and exploitation become more complicated. Lawyers may feel threatened, even exploited, by what I have written. At the same time, however, as a female researcher and a paralegal—a subordinate—I have felt exploited by their attempts to put me in my so-called proper place. Being screamed at, treated as less intelligent, and bullied are not empowering experiences. When we privilege the usual script on ethnographic authority—(white) male as author—these shifting and changing regimes of power in the field are obscured. By contrast, the outlaw position brings these shifts and changes into bold relief. Indeed, it is precisely the multiple and shifting nature of the outlaw position in the field that renders my work empowering to some—"I want my real name in your book," boring to others, and a lethal weapon to still others.

NOTES

1. In Stacey's (1988) influential article, "Can There Be a Feminist Ethnography?" she describes the research process for *Brave New Families*. Here, she concludes that there can only be "ethnographies that are partially feminist [or] accounts of culture [or both] enhanced by the application of feminist perspectives" (p. 26).

2. My research was on litigators. Compared to other specialties within law, litigation has the highest percentage of men, 88% (Menkel-Meadow, 1989).

3. There are two sets of ethical questions related to my fieldwork. The first concerns the issue of covert versus overt fieldwork, which I discuss in the introductory chapter of my book, *Gender Trials: Emotional Lives in Contemporary Law Firms* (Pierce, 1995). The second set of concerns revolves around the more personal ethical dilemmas of the moment. For instance, though I promised confidentiality to my subjects, writing about their personal confidences—even in a disguised form—sometimes felt like betrayal. This chapter focuses on this second set of concerns.

4. See Kondo (1990) for an interesting discussion of how an epiphanal moment in her fieldwork in Japan led her to shift the focus of her study.

5. I am using *regimes of power* in Judith Butler's (1990) sense of the term. Butler rejects the notion that power is simply an exchange between individuals—a constant inversion between oppressor and oppressed. By contrast, she conceptualized power in a Foucaultian sense, wherein power is dispersed through all social relationships. In this sense, power can neither be withdrawn nor refused but only redeployed. Such an understanding highlights the ways that power is diffuse, shifting, and changing.

6. I have used pseudonyms throughout this essay to protect the confidentiality of subjects in this study.

7. Some of the works I had read as a graduate student included William Whyte's (1943/1993) methodological appendix to his classic book, *Streetcorner Society*; McCall and Simmons's (1969) anthology on participant observation; Hughes (1960); and Burgess (1982). Many of the more reflexive works written by feminist scholars that address these issues had not yet been published (e.g., Krieger, 1991; Stacey, 1990; D. Wolf, 1995; M. Wolf, 1992).

The one exception is sociologist Shulamit Reinharz's (1979) book, *On Becoming a Social Scientist*. Although the earlier edition is not explicitly feminist, many of the issues she raised about reflexivity were reintroduced later by sociologists such as Krieger (1991).

8. In Arlie Hochschild's (1983) conception of the term, *emotional labor* requires workers "to induce or suppress feeling in order to sustain the outward countenance that produces the proper state of mind in others" (p. 7). Just as the flight attendants in Hochschild's study were expected to hide feelings of irritation with difficult passengers and display feelings of concern for their welfare, paralegals are expected to be deferential to trial lawyers and to provide emotional support for them. On the other hand, the work of trial lawyers demands not only skills in legal research and writing, but emotional presentations of self as intimidating or strategically friendly.

9. In her book, *Bodies That Matter*, Butler (1993) makes this argument with respect to gay and lesbian activists who have reappropriated the stigmatized term *queer* as a positive and affirmative political identity. Butler suggests, however, that such reappropriations do not always work for progressive political ends.

10. Many paralegals and secretaries I interviewed expressed a critical perspective on the gendered division of labor within law firms. In "Gendering Consent and Resistance in Paralegal Work," I discussed a number of strategies female paralegals employ to resist degradation on the job (Pierce, 1995).

11. In an intriguing article on academic men and feminism, Judith Newton and Judith Stacey (1995) also found that unequal power relations strongly informed their ethnographic encounters.

12. Indeed, in the review of my book, *Gender Trials,* for my tenure case in 1996, one mainstream sociologist noted "Professor Pierce's failure to employ scientific objectivity throughout the manuscript" (Brustein, November 25, 1996, p. 3). And another member of the faculty wrote in the *Majority Report* that "the bitterness expressed in the methodological appendix of the book made him question Professor Pierce's credibility as a researcher." (Majority Report, November 25, 1996).

13. I am using the terms *mainstream sociology* and *positivism* interchangeably.

14. In my research, I found that typical paralegal job descriptions do not list the feminized emotional dimensions of the job. See my discussion of job descriptions in chapter 4, "Mothering Paralegals: Emotional Labor in a Feminized Occupation" (Pierce, 1995).

REFERENCES

Abu-Lughod, L. (1993). *Writing women's worlds: Bedouin stories.* Berkeley: University of California Press.

Austin, R. (1989). Sapphire bound. *Wisconsin Law Review, 3,* 539-578.

Behar, R. (1993). *Translated woman: Crossing the border with Esperanza's story.* Boston: Beacon.

Behar, R. (1995). Writing in my father's name: A diary of *Translated woman*'s first year. In R. Behar & D. Gordon (Eds.), *Women writing culture.* Berkeley: University of California Press.

Blauner, R., & Wellman, D. (1973). Toward the decolonization of social research. In J. Ladner (Ed.), *The death of white sociology* (pp. 310-330). New York: Vintage.

Bornstein, K. (1994). *Gender outlaw: On men, women and the rest of us.* New York: Routledge.

Brustein, W. (1996). Letter to Steven Rosenstone, Professor and Dean of the College of Liberal Arts, University of Minnesota, regarding "Chair's Recommendation for Promotion and Tenure of Professor Jennifer Pierce." Available from Dr. J. Pierce, Sociology Department, University of Minnesota, Minneapolis, MN, 55455.

Burgess, R. (1982). *Field research: A sourcebook and field manual.* London: Unwin.

Butler, J. (1990). *Gender trouble: Feminism and the subversion of identity.* New York: Routledge.

Butler, J. (1993). *Bodies that matter: On the discursive limits of sex.* New York: Routledge.

Cixous, H. (1981). The laugh of Medusa. In E. Marks & I. de Courtivron (Eds.), *New French feminisms* (pp. 90-98). New York: Schocken.

Clifford, J. (1988). *The predicament of culture.* Cambridge, MA: Harvard University Press.

de Beauvoir, S. (1949). *The second sex.* New York: Knopf.

Easton, M. (1994). *Knowing gender in an unknowable world: The possibilities of poststructuralism for research on gender.* Unpublished paper, Department of Sociology, University of Minnesota at Minneapolis.

Freud, S. (1963). *Jokes and their relation to the unconscious.* New York: Norton. (original work published in 1905)

Hertz, R., & Imber, J. B. (1995). *Studying elites using qualitative methods.* Thousand Oaks, CA: Sage.

Hochschild, A. (1983). *The managed heart: Commercialization and human feeling.* Berkeley: University of California Press.

Hughes, E. (1960). Introduction: The place of field work in the social sciences. In B. H. Junker (Ed.), *Fieldwork: An introduction to the social sciences.* Chicago: University of Chicago Press.

Kleinman, S., & Copp, M. (1994). *Emotions and fieldwork* (Qualitative Research Series, No. 28). Thousand Oaks, CA: Sage.

Kondo, D. (1990). Crafting selves: Power, gender and discourse of identity. In *A Japanese workplace.* Chicago: University of Chicago Press.

Krieger, S. (1991). *Social science and the self.* New Brunswick, NJ: Rutgers University Press.

Majority report regarding promotion and tenure of professor Jennifer Pierce. (1996, November 26). Available from Dr. J. Pierce, Sociology Department, University of Minnesota, Minneapolis, MN, 55455.

Mauss, M. (1954). *The gift.* Glencoe, IL: Free Press.

McCall, G., & Simmons, J. (1969). *Issues in participant observation.* New York: Addison-Wesley.

Menkel-Meadow, C. (1989). Feminization of the legal profession: The comparative sociology of women lawyers. In R. Abel & P. Lewis (Eds.), *Lawyers in society: Vol 3. Comparative theories.* Berkeley: University of California Press.

Minh-Ha, T. (1989). *Woman, native, other: Writing, postcoloniality and feminism.* Bloomington: Indiana University Press.

Newton, J., & Stacey, J. (1995). Ms. Representations: Reflections on studying academic men. In R. Behar & D. Gordon (Eds.), *Women writing culture* (pp. 287-305). Berkeley: University of California Press.

Pierce, J. (1995). *Gender trials: Emotional lives in contemporary law firms.* Berkeley: University of California Press.

Rabinow, P. (1977). *Reflections on fieldwork in Morocco.* Berkeley: University of California Press.

Reinharz, S. (1979). *On becoming a social scientist.* San Francisco: Jossey-Bass.

Stacey, J. (1988). Can there be A feminist ethnography? *Women's Studies International Forum, 11,* 21-27.

Stacey, J. (1990). *Brave new families.* New York: Basic Books.

Whyte, W. (1993). *Streetcorner society* (4th ed.). Chicago: University of Chicago Press. (Original work published in 1943)

Wise, S. (1987). A framework of discussing ethical issues in feminist research: A review of the literature. In *Writing feminist biographies: Vol. 2. Using life histories* (Studies in Sexual Politics, No. 19, p. 47-88). Manchester, UK: University of Manchester, Department of Sociology.

Wolf, D. (Ed.). (1995). *Feminist dilemmas in fieldwork.* Boulder, CO: Westview.

Wolf, M. (1992). *A thricetold tale: Feminism, postmodernism and ethnographic responsibility.* Stanford, CA: Stanford University Press.

14

The Place of the Personal and the Subjective in Religious Studies

Rita M. Gross

Religious Studies is an academic discipline devoted to studying and commenting on the extremely diverse religious beliefs and behaviors found in all cultures around the globe, in all periods of human history. Nevertheless, studying or teaching religion in the college or university is also a very politically sensitive enterprise because everyone has personal opinions, often very strong personal opinions, about religion. Because of the intensely personal, often passionate, attitudes people have about religion, calls for neutrality and objectivity can be very strong in this field, and expressing one's own personal interest in or subjective views about religion can be dangerous to one's career (unless one expresses critical, antireligious sentiments). How did this situation develop?

The European enlightenment brought about great changes in how religion was understood, which made possible the eventual emergence of the discipline of religious studies. Rather than being part of a communal ethos, religion came to be viewed as a personal belief system to be studied because of personal religious commitments (or rejected because of personal conclusions—something not really possible in premodern Europe or any other traditional culture). This, in turn, caused changes in how religion was studied, as Christian theology fell from its position as "queen of the sciences" in medieval universities to become a much less prestigious and much less common pursuit. These changes in perspective, though very briefly sketched here, largely explain how studying religion was viewed until relatively recently (the 1950s or 1960s) in the United States, which is my primary reference point in this discussion. Until the 1950s and 1960s, most study of religion was done at private colleges and universities, which often had some Christian denominational affiliation. Studying "religion" really meant studying Christianity. The religious studies requirement common in the graduation requirements of these colleges and universities was defended as a strategy for strengthening the religious affiliations and commitments fostered earlier by churches. All this is in accord with the European enlightenment notion of religion as a personal, private matter, not a public ethos. Meanwhile, in the United States, large public universities not connected in any way with any religious denomination became increasingly important as more and more people received their educations in such institutions rather than in private colleges and universities. And it seemed self-evident to most people that religion could not and should not be taught in any way at such institutions. This too is completely in accord with the European enlightenment notion of religion as a personal, not a public, affair. Most also assumed that to study a religion is synonymous with advocating for that religion. (This has, in fact, been the dominant mode in traditional forms of religion worldwide.) Clearly, if advocacy for a religion were only a method and motive for studying it, public universities devoted to educating people from very diverse backgrounds could not afford the divisiveness religion would have brought to the curriculum.

As an example, when I was an undergraduate at a public university, my formal major was philosophy, despite my interest in religious studies. I was told that to teach about religion in such an institution would violate the separation of church and state and was both impossible and nonsensical. (I did manage nevertheless to study a good bit of what today could easily be taught in any religious studies department.) Eight years after my graduation, I returned to teach religious studies at a different campus of that same university system. But I returned to teach world religions, not only Christianity. Clearly, something major had changed in the meantime, in that particular university system. This change was repeated at countless other institutions, both private and public. Private institutions, which had always taught "religion" now routinely teach world religions, not just Christianity, and the study of religion is no longer so frequently viewed as a way to further inculcate the training of a confirmation class. Public universities now routinely include a department of religious studies. It is assumed by all that this department will teach about all religions, not just Christianity, and it is crucial to such institutions that the teaching of religion not be a front for evangelizing for that religion. What had happened to promote these drastic changes? In answering that question, we will also discover why calls for neutrality and objectivity are so strong in religious studies and why expressing personal interests and subjective views about religion can be so dangerous.

Beginning in the late 19th century, a new discipline had developed, primarily in European universities. Its German title, *religionswissenschaft,* the scientific study of religion, says best what this discipline wanted to accomplish. The transformations regarding the study of religion in universities and colleges in the United States, both public and private, that I just described were largely due to the influence of this European model of how religion should be studied. So it is important to discuss why this new discipline developed and its methods and the ideals involved.

This new field developed in large part because, in the late 19th century, so much new information was being discovered about religion and because this newly discovered information dealt with a multitude of religions, not just Christianity. Whole dead religions of the ancient world came to light again, largely through exploration and archaeology in the Middle East. These discoveries forced new critical historical scholarship about the Bible. At the same time, the wealth of Indian religions and the religious universes of China and Japan were being studied in depth. Last, early anthropologists brought home a veritable cornucopia of religious beliefs, practices, and artifacts that seemed thoroughly exotic and fascinating to Europeans. All these discoveries dramatically changed how Christianity was studied and definitively undercut any Christian claims about its uniqueness and superiority. Suddenly, there was much more to religion than just Christianity, on the one hand, and so-called heathenism on the other. More and more, Christianity came to be seen as another religion among many religions, not as religion per se; this change is a conceptual revolution still contested by many conservative Christians.

For *religionswissenschaft,* religion is global in scope, and Christianity holds no privileged position among religions. Theological and subjective judgments about the *value* of any religion were simply inadmissible, impossible for the *scientific* study of religion. Thus, we see the source of the fact that the study of religion is now practiced, in both public and private colleges and universities, as the *comparative* study of religion, inevitably cross-cultural and global in scope. But we also see the source of the difficulty with expressing any personal or subjective views about religion in the discipline of religious studies.

The proponents of *religionswissenshaft* claimed that they were scientists, not philosophers or theologians, which made their method of studying religion academically rigorous and appropriate in the modern university. To study religion "scientifically" meant to them that they were simply observing religion "objectively," without adding or subtracting anything, just as a scientist observes nature objectively, without any personal interest in or bias about what he or she is observing. Like many 19th-century scholars, they really did believe in such objectivity, in being so able to so divest oneself of one's cultural baggage that it disappeared completely. If one couldn't attain that ideal 100%, one should at least keep trying. This was not a situation that created much room for talking about the personal and the subjective in religious studies. Instead, it created a lot of what I call *science envy*. Claims about the possibility of such objectivity still seem self-evident and unproblematic to many contemporary scholars of religion. The strictest of the *religionswissenschaft* proponents also claim that theirs is the *only* legitimate method for studying religion, at least in the academy. Academic studies of religion must not be tainted with anything personal or subjective, evaluative or normative, because such studies are not knowledge but only opinion. This claim also contributes to the science envy so apparent in some aspects of religious studies and is also still held by many scholars of religion. But the weakness, indeed the untenableness, of these two claims is the wedge that reintroduces the possibility of academically respectable expressions of personal interest and subjective judgments about religions into our discipline. The necessarily and inherently comparative character of our discipline, however, is incontestable.

The historical narrative just outlined has led to the current tangled situation in the field of religious studies. Theology, understood broadly as the actual claims regarding the nature of reality made by religions, has, of course, not gone away, and people still do take religions to be personally relevant. If one is going to study a religion, then one cannot avoid studying its theology. It is impossible to teach a course on world religions without teaching about myriad truth claims made by religions. How do you do so within the value system of *religion-swisssenschaft*? The solution was to have outsiders teach religions. That was thought to be much safer, because outsiders would be neutral and objective about a religious system, whereas insiders could not be objective and might describe the religion positively and persuasively. For Hinduism and Buddhism, that was very easy to do; until very recently, these religions were most often studied and taught by Westerners who were not themselves Hindus or Buddhists. But it's much harder to have Judaism and Christianity taught by genuine outsiders. It seems that not enough Asian non-Christians were interested in or allowed to receive the training required to teach Judaism or Christianity in Western universities. So Judaism and Christianity have been taught by nominal Jews and Christians who were expected to do historical scholarship and to be disinterested in the religion itself. It was thought to be safer to entrust the study of religion to atheists and unbelievers, who were thought to be more objective and neutral. (That atheism or unbelief is itself a religious position was ignored or not recognized by these advocates of neutrality.) The strange effect of this logic is that so-called objectivity and neutrality actually mean *caring against religion rather than caring for religion* (O'Flaherty, 1988, p. 18), because complete indifference to the claims made by religions is impossible. But one set of reactions—caring against—is promoted as preferable to the other set of reactions—caring for—as if it were more neutral, more objective. It's a very strange situation when one of the best ways to further claims to academic rigor is to say one has no *personal* interest in what one spends one's life studying, without getting paid a whole lot for it!

But what about someone who is actually interested in religious truth claims and practices spiritual disciplines according to some of these teachings? Under the claims of orthodox science of religion, such a person could not be a good scholar because such a scholar is not neutral vis-a-vis religion. This has led to a lot of hypocrisy, as some scholars actually do practice the religions they study but do so secretly. This conundrum has been particularly difficult in one of the areas in which I had done much of my work—Buddhist studies. I was one of the first "out" Buddhist scholars of religion and have done a lot of Buddhist feminist reconstructive work (Gross, 1993, 1998) for which I am well known. A friend of mine was interviewing a young graduate student on the job market last fall. She asked her about her approach to the study of religion; when she heard the replies, she said, "Oh, it sounds as if you've been influenced by Rita Gross." "Not me; her practice of Buddhism obscures her ability to understand it." I would reply that my practice of Buddhism has certainly changed my understanding of Buddhism but not so as to make Buddhism more obscure, either to me or to those to whom I explain it.

According to some in religious studies, the way out of this illogical impasse is to admit the impossibility of complete objectivity and neutrality and the inevitability of a subjective and personal element, not only in the study of religion but in all studies. Open admission of the obvious, that our personal interests and standpoints do influence our choices of subject matter, the data we see, and the conclusions we derive, does not turn us into unbalanced, fanatical zealots and proselytizers. Nor does it mean we become sloppy scholars; good rules of argument and good use of evidence remain important. But we do become more honest—and more humble, which, though considered a virtue, is not often something to which scholars are prone.

As teachers, we should always make it clear that teaching about religion is not the same as giving religious instruction in the classroom. We do not give religious instruction in our classrooms, though we can let our students know that we have interests and preferences regarding religion, for which we can make sound arguments. For example, it would be very difficult for me to teach religious studies without my feminist stance coming through clearly. But none of my exams or essay assignments require a feminist stance on the part of the student, though they may well be required to demonstrate that they understand the arguments made by feminists in religion. Much as in teaching evolution, still a touchy topic in some universities, we require students to learn the arguments, and we test them on how well they understand the arguments regarding a certain position, but we don't test their personal beliefs.

Actually, the issue of the personal and the subjective plays out differently in the two major subdivisions within religious studies. The first of these is the descriptive study of religion, devoted to historical and anthropological interests (which describes *what is* concerning religious beliefs and behaviors). The second is the normative or constructive study of religion, devoted to theology and ethics (which studies claims about the nature of reality and what *should be,* regarding religious beliefs and behaviors and often enters the debates concerning what "should be"). Religious studies journals and departments argue endlessly about the relationship between these two wings of the discipline. Some claim that they are completely distinct and separate; some scholars who take this position often also argue that religious studies should consist only of descriptive enterprises, that any normative or constructive concerns are invalid and inappropriate. It is no surprise that scholars in this camp also argue most vociferously that objectivity and neutrality are possible and desirable. Others, myself included, see inevitable links between descriptive and normative studies in religion, arguing that part of the job description of a scholar of religious studies includes evaluating religious phenomena and discussing what religious beliefs and behaviors are more likely to promote human and planetary well-being (Gross, 1993, 1996). Needless to say, those of us who take this position regarding the field of religious studies are not so afraid of or worried about the personal and the subjective in religious studies because we claim that they are impossible to avoid, even in descriptive dimensions of the field.

The case for admitting the subjective and personal in the descriptive wing of religious studies turns on claims that the scholar inevitably brings his or her own outlook, his or her experience, training, life situation, and values into the study, making objectivity and neutrality impossible. One cannot get completely outside one's skin and one's culture to observe religion from some neutral nowhere, reporting what is, completely separate from one's own observing viewpoint. That being the case, claims to pure objectivity only obscure the dense interplay between "what is" and "what I see" in descriptions of religious phenomena, making "what is" less, not more, evident. Scholars are not simply blank receptive mirrors on which can be inscribed the data of the religious situation they are studying. They also project onto the data from their subjectivity. The more adamant the claims that this process is not occurring, the more the data are actually skewed and obscured. The only correctives are self-consciousness and self-awareness, and the modesty to admit that one may not be seeing everything. Then, what one does see and report on will be much more accurate.

In my view, the back of the claim that descriptive studies in religion could be completely objective was broken by women's studies scholarship in religion. Women studies scholarship has demonstrated, beyond any doubt, that who the scholar is determines, in part, what the scholar sees. Before the second wave of feminism, the study of religion was almost exclusively in the hands of men—and what they saw was the religious activities and thinking of other men. When I entered graduate school in religious studies in 1965, there were only 12 women in a student body of over 400 at the University of Chicago Divinity School, and people were worried that so many women (six in the entering class) were pursuing graduate studies in religion. It was no surprise, given this situation, we students were taught *only* about what men did and thought religiously. Women were literally invisible to these male scholars. If they ever studied anything about women, it was not what women themselves thought or did but what men thought about and did with women. So even when peripherally studying women, they were still really studying men, while also claiming to be doing objective and value-free scholarship. These male scholars were quite unaware of their androcentrism, of the way in which they projected onto the data their own deeply held viewpoint that men were more interesting, important, and *normal* than women. They simply did not notice that half the participants of any religion would be women and that often, cultural norms dictated that women's religious lives would be considerably different from men's. This failure to study women, when infrequently pointed out, was excused by the claim that women were subservient and secondary in most religious situations. Somehow, in their minds, women's subservience meant that a complete and accurate portrayal of the religion they were studying could be obtained even while ignoring women.

Their claims to objective, value-free scholarship turned into ridicule of the first feminist scholars, who pointed out that androcentric scholarship provided an incomplete, skewed, and inaccurate portrait of the religion being studied. Ridicule turned into resistance to feminists' demonstrations that studying women's religious lives changed the reported portrait considerably. That resistance generated negative consequences for these feminist scholars, who were often denied good jobs and career advancement by androcentric scholars who discredited their work, often claiming that it lacked objectivity or was biased because it focused on women. All these value judgments made by androcentric scholars—because of their androcentric outlook and values—would have been less problematic if they had been able to admit that they simply regarded men as more interesting, important, and normal than women and, therefore, focused their attentions on men. But that seemingly obvious fact was adamantly denied. *Obvious selection of data based on one's own values and interests combined with the illusion of objectivity is an especially pernicious and dangerous combination.*

Feminist scholarship in religion has demonstrated far more than that who a person is often greatly influences what a scholar sees and what that scholar finds interesting and important. Feminist scholarship has also demonstrated that including women in the data has a greater impact on our understanding of religions than simply providing add-on information. As I wrote when discussing this point in my book, *Feminism and Religion—An Introduction* (Gross, 1996),

Feminist scholars often discover that information about women simply cannot be added onto the picture scholars already have. *In almost all cases, they discover that they have to repaint the whole picture,* which . . . is much more troublesome . . . than merely filling in some details in a blank corner of the canvas. (p. 76)

This is the case not only in religious studies but in virtually all disciplines. Feminist scholars, who were propelled into the study of women by our own personal experiences as women in a male-dominated field and confess our personal standpoints and interests, have produced scholarship that has considerably changed the whole academy in the past 25 years (Kramarae & Spender, 1992).

The field of religious studies has only reluctantly accepted feminists scholars' demonstrations that the standpoint and interests of the scholar affect scholarship. But more recently, another perspective demonstrating the same claim has become quite popular, especially in comparative studies of South Asian religions, Hinduism in particular. This is the postcolonial critique, which claims that the common portrait of Hinduism found in virtually every world religions textbook, as well as in much of the advanced scholarship about Hinduism, exists much more in the minds of Western (male) observers of Hinduism than in the lives of the vast majority of ordinary Hindus.

This Western version of Hinduism, it is claimed, was actually the product of one male educated elite (Western) talking to another educated male elite (Hindu). It focused on ancient texts (the *Vedas* and *Upanishads*) that are barely known by the vast majority of Hindus, but that are important to this small male elite with classical educations (Sangari & Vaid, 1989). It ignores the fact that much Hindu religiosity is focused on rituals rather than texts and that for most Hindus, taking *darshan* (auspicious seeing) of an icon or a teacher is far more important than reading or hearing a text. (But because Western religions are text based, Western observers were far more likely to notice textual dimensions of Hinduism, even if they are a minor strand in the whole fabric of Hinduism.) Because the ancient texts favored by Western scholars, the *Upanishads* in particular, teach a highly abstract monistic philosophy in which deity is nonexistent or unimportant, generations of Western undergraduates in world religions courses have learned that Hinduism is a monistic philosophy, whereas the vast majority of Hindus worship the various deities of the Hindu pantheon with ecstatic fervor unrivaled in any other religion. If the deities of Hinduism are discussed, one would gain the impression that male deities are the popular norm, and goddesses represent a minor strand of Hindu theism. But if anything is, various versions of the Goddess are the dominant deity of Hinduism. (It has been particularly hard for Western scholars of religion to notice that male monotheism is a peculiarly Western phenomenon unknown in all other religious contexts.) Last, because women were rigorously excluded from text-based dimensions of Hinduism, the religious lives of women were completely ignored. One easily gained the impression that women simply did not participate in the Hindu religion, whereas women carry on richly developed religious lives of their own, separate from male religious specialists and men in general (Falk & Gross, 1989). On this point, the postcolonial and the feminist critiques converge.

But why did early Western observers of Hinduism see a monistic, text-based, male-dominant religion when India presents so much and such overwhelming evidence of ritual, mythology, icon veneration, ecstatic devotionalism, and women's independent religious lives, even in spite of the views of India's educated male elite? Why was it so convenient to have one male elite talk to another male elite while ignoring the everyday Hinduisms that teemed all around them? The postcolonial analysts claim that the conventional Western portrait of Hinduism served the colonial powers very well. For this portrait of Hinduism also included a thesis about Hindu development: the Hinduism of the *Vedas* and *Upanishads* was said to represent so-called true Hinduism, whereas contemporary popular Hinduisms, with their wildly exuberant mythology, rituals, and visual imagery, were a degeneration. Hinduism had fallen on hard times throughout its long history and needed help to revert to its former rational monism. Enter the colonialists and their missionary friends, who were only too glad to criticize contemporary popular Hinduism and offer to replace it with something they deemed more worthy. Thus, the colonial rulers of India gained some moral legitimacy for their occupation of India because of what scholars told them about the development and current status of Hinduism.

Based on my own knowledge of and experience with Hinduism, I would agree that there is no question that the standard portrayal of Hinduism found in Western textbooks bears almost no resemblance to the Hinduism one commonly encounters in India. Clearly, the philosophical and textual preferences of early Western observers of Hinduism were projected onto Hinduism itself, obscuring the myriad phenomena that did not fit into that model of religion. As with androcentric scholars, their ideology that scholarship should be objective and neutral did not protect these scholars from their own subjectivity. To later generations of scholars or scholars from another culture or scholars with a different set of experiences, their subjectivity is glaringly obvious, just as the androcentric subjectivity of the male scholars who dominated religious studies until recently is very obvious to feminist scholars.

The subjectivity of these scholars is itself not so much of a problem because of its inevitability. The damage is done by denial of one's own subjectivity, of one's own standpoint. As we have seen in both examples of unacknowledged subjectivity on the part of the scholar, this denial is especially problematic when the power of the scholar as male or as colonial undercuts and dismisses other subjectivities. Thus, the justification for seeking or claiming objectivity—that it would produce more accurate descriptive scholarship than scholarship that openly admitted its subjective and personal elements—turns out to be quite misleading and very oppressive. When *we*—whatever subjectivity that might be—insist that our subjectivity is normative and neutral, all that results is the constriction of knowledge and oppression of other subjectivities—not objectivity.

But if objectivity and neutrality are impossible simply because there is no neutral "nowhere" from which to conduct one's observations, because personal experiences of gender, class, race, culture, and education inevitably affect what one sees, does that mean we have permission simply to let go of our critical faculties and see what we would like to see? Commentaries from oppressed groups often fall prey to this tendency, as can readily be seen in some fanciful feminist reconstructions of the ancient past. But, obviously, I am not suggesting that because our personal subjectivity inevitably influences what we are interested in and what we see, we can, therefore, ignore research and critical thinking. If anything, because our critical thinking tells us that personal subjectivity always affects scholarship, we should engage in more self-correction and greater modesty. We do not claim that we feminist scholars, for example, now have *the* complete accurate picture, but only that our subjective urgency to know about women's religious lives and to understand women better has improved our understanding of religion in general, has made it more accurate and complete than was possible when all the scholars wore androcentric-colored glasses. Therefore, we should welcome a variety of standpoints and perspectives on our subject matter because such variety will bring us a fuller, richer picture than any single angle of vision. Last, although scholars who long for neutrality and objectivity might regard the inevitable subjectivity of scholarship as a handicap, we can celebrate the creativity that can result when we speak genuinely out of our subjectivity.

Constructive or normative studies in religion have a somewhat different perspective on the place of the personal and subjective in scholarship. On the one hand, by definition, constructive studies evaluate religious phenomena and recommend some alternatives over others. Therefore, they do not claim to be an objective description of what is but a prescription for what should be. As such, the critical thinking of the scholar is paramount in constructive studies in religion. But, on the other hand, constructive theology often expresses significant reluctance to openly admit the importance of personal experience in forming one's theological outlook. Instead, the conventional tendency has been to presume that pure reason, devoid of the influence of one's own life experiences, is the prime mover in theological thinking. In fact, conventionally, the dominant opinion has been that one should rise above and ignore personal, idiosyncratic experience when thinking normatively and should try to achieve a "universal" perspective instead. In addition, theologies often make the claim that their content is not even a human construction at all, but that divine revelation is the ultimate source of the basic ideas and norms of theology. Therefore, it is sometimes argued that such theological givens are unalterable by humans. Clearly, if that were the case, personal experience would be irrelevant to theology. Thus, despite the fact that constructive studies in religion do not claim to be objective and neutral descriptions, nevertheless, they have almost as much difficulty admitting the legitimacy of the genuinely personal and subjective as do descriptive studies.

As in descriptive studies in religion, the first major inroads into the hegemony of impersonal, so-called universal norms in theology were made by feminists, by those of us who were outsiders to the supposedly universal presuppositions of theology. As outsiders, as people who were different, we clearly saw how limited the universal presuppositions of theology were, how much they depended on projections of gender onto conceptualizations of ultimate reality, and how much those projections served the interests and needs of those who had controlled the theologizing process. Paralleling early insights in descriptive studies in religion, much of the early insistence that theology cannot help being personal and subjective was the result of seeing clearly just how androcentric the conventional, supposedly universal theological norms and constructs actually were. Also paralleling conclusions reached by feminist scholars of descriptive studies in religion, feminist theologians claimed that because we cannot avoid subjective elements in our theologizing, we might as well openly admit our guiding experiences and perspectives and use them to further our creative insights. Therefore, feminist theology is unapologetically personal and subjective; in fact, it glories in the openly personal and subjective, combined with rigorous critical thinking. Feminist theology is considerably more up open and up-front in its declarations about the centrality of the personal and subjective in theology than are most feminist scholars who focus on descriptive studies in religion. With this agenda clearly stated, feminist theology has become a major player, especially in Christian and Jewish circles, though it is much less developed in other major world religions.

Noticing how androcentric conventional universal theology actually is, feminist theologians have taken as their first principle the claim that all religious thought is grounded in and derives from human experience. The words and concepts of religion do not come from extrahuman divine sources but from the familiar features of our ordinary human lives. For example, only a society that included the institution of kingship would conceptualize deity as a king, lord, or ruler. Likewise, only a society that prizes the patrilineal relationship between father and son above all other relationships would imagine deity in terms of a father-son relationship. And regarding one of the topics most explored by feminist theology, only a society that regards men as more important, interesting, and normal than women would evaluate an anthropomorphic male deity as acceptable and commonplace while evaluating female anthropomorphic deities as abhorrent and abnormal. Theology is thus always extremely subjective, though that reality is often hidden and denied.

Based on this first principle, feminist theology takes as its second principle the claim that valid theology would reflect and be based on all humans' experiences, not those of a small and limited group of humans. Thus, the express purpose of feminist theology is to reflect on the received norms and insights of the tradition in the light of women's experiences, rejecting and recasting as necessary. In this task, there is no apology for open inclusion of the personal and subjective. In fact, autobiographical elements are quite common in feminist theology, as feminist theologians explore and explain how their formative experiences helped shape their theological outlooks. The common justification for such personal disclosure is that it makes clear and unambiguous what is obscured and hidden in theology without personal disclosure.

Since the rise of feminist theology, many other subjectivities have given themselves permission to speak openly and have taken up the task of articulating their perspectives theologically. Race, class, culture, and sexual orientation are now commonly explored as significant factors that shape one's theology. Even white male heterosexual theologians, who used to think of themselves as so generic, so much the universal norm that admitting their subjectivity was unnecessary, are beginning to explore and express the impact of their personal experiences on their theologies. The result of this celebration of subjectivity in theology is that many more points of view are now expressed, read, and commented on than in earlier, more monolithic times. This can only represent an improvement in theological discourse, as well as an improvement in our recognition and appreciation of human diversity.

Needless to say, just as in descriptive studies, acknowledging the subjective and personal factors in theologizing does not lead to wanton, self-indulgent, narcissistic self-expression. Theological thinking is always a process of interaction between the received tradition and the reflecting theologian. That process requires deep knowledge of the tradition and keenly critical thinking, and these are clearly present in all the new theologies. What is different with the new so-called subjective theologies of identity—feminist, womanist (black women's theology), black, Asian, Asian American, Latina, gay, lesbian, and so on—is the sheer variety of viewpoints from which theologizing is done and the honesty and openness with which the subjective and the personal in theology is disclosed.

Unfortunately, in North America, the situation I am describing for normative studies pertains almost exclusively to those who do constructive work out of a Jewish or a Christian perspective. The academy has learned how to accommodate Jews and Christians who think normatively, but because of the confusion regarding the relationship between teaching or studying a religion and practicing a religion discussed at the beginning of this chapter, the bias remains that all religions except Judaism and Christianity should be approached only descriptively, preferably by outsiders. In other words, the legitimacy of the constructive or normative study of religion is denied for any religions except Judaism and Christianity. For complex reasons, in the cases of Confucianism, Taoism, and Islam, many East Asians and many Muslims do, in fact, research and teach these religions, making the prohibition against the personal and the subjective in the study of these religions less stringent. But the native speakers of these traditions rarely do genuinely constructive theology; they study the received theological tradition instead. Thus the issue I am addressing, that of the difficulties faced by those of us with normative interests in religions other than Christianity and Judaism, is not corrected by the ease with which East Asian and Muslim scholars are admitted to the academy.

As a result, other religions, especially Hinduism and Buddhism, are usually taught and researched only descriptively, as if they were archaic museum pieces foreign to North Americans and irrelevant to the modern world. Unlike Judaism or Christianity, they are not taught or studied as living wisdom traditions that are still developing in response to modernity or as possible gold mines of inspiration for *us* for dealing with contemporary crises. This is an unfortunate and artificial situation; there is no cogent reason why the Asian and indigenous wisdom traditions should be so circumscribed in religious studies or why they should be approached so differently from Judaism and Christianity. In addition, unfortunately, a scholar who takes a constructive approach to Buddhism or Hinduism is in great jeopardy. In fact, nowhere is expression of the subjective and the personal in religious studies so repressed and so dangerous to one's career as it is for those of us with constructive interests in Buddhism and Hinduism. There are few places to publish research on such topics because of the editorial policies of journals and publishers. A track record of such constructive work in Buddhism or Hinduism means that one is perceived as fitting nowhere—neither in positions devoted to Asian religions, which are reserved for translators and historians, not constructive thinkers, nor in positions devoted to theology and constructive studies in religions, which almost by definition are reserved for Christians or, more rarely, Jews.

This final barrier to admitting that personal and subjective elements are an inevitable and legitimate dimension of religious studies has yet to be overcome. Those involved in descriptive studies of religion are admitting, somewhat reluctantly, that who the scholar is influences what the scholar sees and what conclusions he or she draws. Jewish and Christian constructive thinkers have learned how to do theology without the kind of exclusive advocacy that is so inappropriate for the academy; they have also become much more comfortable admitting the personal sources of their theologies, and the academy has learned how to find a place for such thinkers. But what about the scholar with constructive interests in some other religion than Judaism or Christianity, especially those with normative interests in Buddhism and Hinduism?

In conclusion, I have argued throughout this chapter that subjective and personal elements in the study of religion are inevitable. Therefore, it does no good to advocate the impossible goals of neutrality and objectivity. Scholarship will be much more adequate if we properly understand the role of the personal and the subjective in religious studies. But especially because of the power of religion in human life and the dangers of religious advocacy, accommodating the influence of the personal and the subjective is probably more sensitive and delicate in religious studies than in many other disciplines.

I believe that several guidelines are essential to accommodating inevitable personal and subjective influences in religious studies without allowing them to degenerate into advocacy and dogmatism. The first of these guidelines is always to maintain a comparative dimension in religious studies. The founder of the discipline of the academic study of religion, Max Muller (as quoted in Paden, 1988), is famous for his slogan, "To know one religion is to know none" (p. 38). He is certainly correct. And the more we delve into personal interests in religion, the more necessary it is to maintain the perspective and the corrective provided by the "comparative mirror" (p. 164), whether we are doing descriptive or normative scholarship. When we are genuinely, wholeheartedly comparative in our study of religion, it is virtually impossible to become intolerant, narrow advocates for our subjectively generated approaches to religion and our personal agendas with religion. When we are genuinely, wholeheartedly comparative in our studies of religion, we cannot help but see that there are a multiplicity of other possible ways than our own to think, to live, and to practice religion.

Second, I would argue that the study of religion is vastly improved by admitting the validity of diverse methods and encouraging all of them. This position is greatly preferable to the methodological straitjacket found especially in some descriptive approaches to religion. For example, in the field of Buddhist studies, translation and historical studies are often considered to be the only legitimate methods with which to study Buddhism; the study of contemporary Buddhism or understandings of Buddhism that include personal experience of the Buddhist lifestyle are simply not admitted into the academic arena. In other cases, there might be promotion of deconstruction, for example, to the denigration of all other theological methods. Or in feminist theology, one often encounters the bias that only post-Christian feminist spirituality is genuinely feminist, that feminists who remain within the framework of a traditional religion have simply been co-opted by patriarchy. But the study of religion requires translators, historians, field workers, constructive thinkers, insiders, outsiders . . . Some of these methods give freer rein to the subjective and personal than do others. But the field is richer and our understanding of religion deeper if, as professional students of religion, we encourage methodological flexibility and variety.

Those who are less prone to use methods that encourage subjective, personal explorations of religion will rein in those of us who are more prone to personal and subjective explorations if we slip into inappropriate advocacy in our personal commentaries on religion. Conversely, when those who are less prone to take account of the fact that religion is existentially relevant make sweeping claims for their methods, those of us who revel in religions' subjective significance can tweak them into realizing that without people who practice religion and care about it, they would have nothing to study; there would be no religions. Last, no matter what methods we prefer or what religions we study, we should always know who we are and who we are not and be completely candid about it. We should not pretend to an objectivity and neutrality that are impossible nor to a universalism that is arrogant.

REFERENCES

Falk, N. A., & Gross, R. M. (1989). *Unspoken worlds: Women's religious lives.* Belmont, CA: Wadsworth.

Gross, R. M. (1993). *Buddhism after patriarchy: A feminist history, analysis, and reconstruction of Buddhism.* Albany, NY: State University of New York Press.

Gross, R. M. (1996). *Feminism and religion: An introduction.* Boston: Beacon.

Gross, R. M. (1998). *Soaring and settling: Buddhist perspectives on contemporary social and religious issues.* New York: Continuum.

Kramarae, C., & Spender, D. (1992). *The knowledge explosion: Generations of feminist scholarship.* New York: Teachers College Press.

O'Flaherty, W. D. (1988). *Other peoples' myths.* New York: Macmillan.

Paden, W. E. (1988). *Religious worlds: The comparative study of religion.* Boston: Beacon.

Sangari, K., & Vaid, S. (Eds.). (1989). *Recasting women: Essays in colonial history.* New Delhi: Kali for Women.

Index

About the Contributors

Miriam E. Cameron, RN, PhD, is Center Associate at the Center for Bioethics at the University of Minnesota-Minneapolis. She has an MA in Philosophy, an MS in Psychiatric-Mental Health Nursing, and a PhD in Nursing from the University of Minnesota. An author, researcher, teacher, and consultant about bioethics, she has published books, journal articles, book chapters, news articles, and columns about bioethics, including the book, *Living with AIDS: Experiencing Ethical Problems.* Formerly Assistant Editor and columnist on legal and ethical issues for the *Journal of Professional Nursing,* she is currently the Ethics Editor for the *Journal of Nursing Law.* She is currently conducting cross-cultural research and writing about her ethics research.

Margaret A. Diekemper, RNC, MSN, is Assistant Professor of Nursing at Maryville University and Community Health Nurse Specialist at the Vietnamese Immigrant Health Center, both in St. Louis, Missouri. She received her undergraduate and graduate nursing degrees from St. Louis University. She serves as a manuscript reviewer for *Public Health Nursing.* Along with coauthors Drake and SmithBattle, she has been funded for a two-phase interpretive research process on community health nursing practice and expertise.

Mary Ann Drake, PhD, RN, is Associate Professor of Nursing at Webster University, St. Louis, Missouri. She received her undergraduate degree from Corpus Christi State University in Texas and both her graduate and doctoral degrees from St. Louis University. Along with SmithBattle and Diekemper, she has been funded for a two-phase interpretive resarch process on community health nursing practice and expertise.

Kimberly D. Elsbach, PhD, is Assistant Professor of Management at the Graduate School of Management at the University of California, Davis. Her research focuses on the perception and management of individual and organizational images, identities, and reputations. Her work has been published in a number of scholarly outlets, including *Administrative Science Quarterly, Academy of Management Journal,* and *Organization.* Her study of impression management in the California cattle industry won the 1993 Louis R. Pondy Award for Best Paper from a Dissertation, from the Organization and Management Theory Division of the Academy of Management. She is currently on the editorial board of *Administrative Science Quarterly* and *Organizational Research Methods.*

Marie F. Gates, PhD, RN, is Associate Professor at the University of Missouri-Kansas City, School of Nursing. She has conducted qualitative research in the following interest areas: care and cure experiences of persons who were dying in hospital and hospice settings, caregiving and carereceiving experiences of African American women with breast cancer, and youngsters who give care to adult family members with cancer and other chronic illnesses. She has also participated in the Michigan Oral History Project in which career interviews of renowned public health nursing leaders were collected. Her undergraduate, graduate, and doctoral degrees were received from Wayne State University in Detroit, Michigan.

Rita M. Gross, PhD is Professor Emerita at the University of Wisconsin-Eau Claire, having earned her doctorate from the University of Chicago. She is the author of *Feminism and Religion, Buddhism after Patriarchy: A Feminist History, Analysis, and Reconstruction of Buddhism,* and *Soaring and Settling: Buddhist Perspectives on Contemporary Social and Religious Issues.* She coedited, with Nancy Auer Falk, *Unspoken Worlds: Women's Religious Lives,* now in its third edition. With Terry Muck, she coedited *Buddhists Talk About Jesus; Christians Talk About the Buddha.* She is coeditor of *The Buddhist-Christian Studies Journal* and a contributing editor to *the Journal of Feminist Studies in Religion.* She has written numerous articles on methodology in the study of religion, Buddhist-Christian dialogue, women and Buddhism, women in world religions, and feminist theology.

Pamela S. Hinds, PhD, RN, CS, is Coordinator of Nursing Research and Associate Director of Research for Behavioral Medicine at St. Jude Children's Research Hospital. She is the chair of the Nursing Research Committee for the Pediatric Oncology Group and a member of the Association of Pediatric Oncology Association, the Oncology Nursing Society, Sigma Theta Tau International, Sigma Xi, and The American Nurses Association. She has conducted research